AROMATHERAPY STEP BY STEP

A simple step by step, easy to follow guide which explains the principles and applications of Aromatherapy

AROMATHERAPY
STEP BY STEP

Published by

Douglas Barry Publications

First Floor Suite,
253 Selhurst Road
South Norwood
London
SE25 6XP
ENGLAND

Tel 020 8680 9631
E-mail dbarrypubs@aol.com

FIRST PUBLISHED IN THE U.K. 1992

AROMATHERAPY
STEP BY STEP
REVISED SECOND EDITION 1999

COPYRIGHT 1992, 1999
©RENÉE TANNER

British Library - A CIP Catalogue
record for this book is available
from the British Library.

I.S.B.N.   0-9516203-6-3

ACKNOWLEDGEMENTS

I am indebted to my family for all the time, energy and constant encouragement given me during the writing of the manuscript.

My thanks to Russell for his endless patience in the preparation of this work. Julie Pankhurst for her attention to detail and constructive suggestions. To my clients, friends and students, both past and present who encouraged me to put my ideas down on paper and without whom this book might never have been written. To my niece Brenda who, despite many operations and the resultant long stays in hospital, has always proven to be nothing short of an inspiration to me and to Diane for her tireless stream of practical suggestions.

In particular, Edward Morrison, my friend of long standing, deserves to be noted for the excellent works of art produced to enhance the profile of each oil.

Finally to readers of my past works whose letters of support, query and question convinced me of the necessity for this new and revised edition.

NOTE TO THE READER

This book is not intended as a substitute for professional or medical advice.

Neither the author nor publisher can accept any responsibility whatsoever for any health problem which results from the use of the methods described in this book.

The reader is urged to consult a general medical practitioner as to the cause or nature of a health problem of any sort.

THE AUTHOR

My own interest in complementary therapy and in particular Aromatherapy, derives from my childhood experience growing up in the Irish countryside. There I was surrounded by nature, herbs, plants and animals. Everyone in those days looked to nature before considering medical intervention from the village doctor.

I spent many afternoons with the village elders observing and taking part in the preparation of lotions and potions. I was privileged to be supported by my grandmother who kept a large kitchen garden and larder of herbal surprises, and a mother who seemed to know the benefits of all that grew.

While most of my compatriots enjoyed sport or other after school activities I collected such goodies as wild strawberries, blackberries, nuts, sloes, apples, etc., anything that could be used for food or treatments.

I spent time helping my mother look after my younger brothers and sisters, which was a very good grounding in caring and learning responsibility. With this background it is not surprising that I should later qualify as a beauty therapist, a complementary therapist and then a teacher.

I have shared my knowledge through running professional training courses at my own and other schools and universities, and giving lectures. Writing seemed a natural progression, so in 1992 I was again fortunate, I had my first Aromatherapy book published.

My students, friends and family have encouraged me to update my Aromatherapy Step by Step book and the aim of this edition remains the same, to provide information for the student and therapist of Aromatherapy. Hence I give you this edition.

Renée

WHAT IS AROMATHERAPY?

When we speak of Aromatherapy we are not talking just about massage but of the various methods and uses of essential oils for the good of the recipient. The oils are obtained from flowers, leaves, plants and trees.

Aroma is taken to mean 'sweet smelling' and therapy suggests 'intent to heal'. The Aromatherapist uses essential oils blended in a base /carrier oil. The blend will depend on the condition being treated, the age of the client and their general wellbeing (blending varies depending on age, condition or illness).

It is important before using essential oils that the properties are known, (e.g. antiseptic) as some oils can be harmful to use in certain conditions; some can even be skin irritants and some may be phototoxic. Just because they are natural doesn't mean they are completely safe and harmless.

The powerful therapeutic healing properties of the oils are used for Aromatherapy in many ways but principally in massage, compress, inhalation, vaporisation and baths.

AN HOLISTIC THERAPY

The word 'holistic' is taken from the Greek word 'holos' which means whole. In Aromatherapy we use it to suggest treatment that takes into account the whole person; mind, body and spirit.

Plato, in his wisdom said, "The cure of the part should not be attempted without treatment of the whole".

The Greek psychologist Carl Jung wrote, "The form an illness takes can be a reflection of a mental state".

I believe that mind, body and spirit are interrelated and whatever affects one will affect the whole. Therefore, it is important before embarking on a treatment that we look at the life and lifestyle of the person being treated.

WHAT ARE ESSENTIAL OILS?
WHAT ARE THEY MADE OF?

Essential oil is a complex substance extracted from a plant. The substance contains the greatest part of the therapeutic properties of the plant though not necessarily all of them.

Plants have naturally occurring volatile, organic constituents. When the relevant part of the plant is subjected to certain processes an aromatic essence is produced commonly referred to as essential oil. The essence occurs naturally in plants at very low concentrations, most vary between 0.1% and 1.0% with a few concentrations as low as 0.01 %. When the essence is extracted and bottled as pure essential oil the concentration is 100%. At this concentration its potency is 100 times stronger than in the natural state.

Each essential oil is made up of different organic molecules. The aromatic and therapeutic properties of each essential oil depends on the combination and concentration of these molecules which belong to several different chemical families including the following:- Acids, Alcohols, Aldehydes, Esters, Keytones, Phenols, Terpenes and many more, including some yet to be discovered; in fact chemists are still unable to reconstitute some essential oils with complete accuracy. It should be noted that the plant's genetic make-up dictates the final composition of the oil.

Any variation due to weather conditions, the time of day or night the plant has been harvested, the soil and altitude at which the plant has been grown will cause some variations to the final essential oil. As with wines there are good and bad years, but of course the oil should always be recognisable as being that of the plant to which it is specific.

The compounds which go to make up the oil are produced in special cells called secretory cells. The cells are grouped together to form the secretory glands which store the oil; some plants have a secretory sac or duct for storage. The secretory cells can be found in almost any part of the plant, e.g. leaves, flowers, bark, fruits, roots, stems or seeds.

Some plants even produce different oils in different parts of the same plant; one such example being the orange tree:

> from the petals we get Neroli.
> from the leaves we get Petitgrain
> from the orange we get Orange.

It is important for all users of essential oil to know the part of the plant used to obtain the oil, as there may be differences in the therapeutic effect of oils from different parts of the same plant. For example Juniper oil produced from the berry is superior to that produced from the leaves of the plant.

Oils have a characteristic odour which changes as the oils volatilize; different components in the oil have different volatilities. Some components are known as "top notes" when the odour disappears relatively quickly, some are known as "middle notes" when the odour lasts longer and those oils with the longest lasting odour are known as base notes.

Although we talk of oils, essential oils are different from all other types of oil in that they are not a fatty substance. Essential oils are not readily soluble in water but some are soluble in alcohol, and almost all in vegetable and mineral oil.

The fact that the oils are naturally occurring does not render them risk free, and misuse can cause serious adverse reactions.
Essential oils are: Volatile, Flammable and Odoriferous.

For safety sake it is worth bearing in mind that to use the full botanical/latin name of the required oil is quite important in order to avoid any misunderstandings. It is also worthwhile confirming with the supplier that the oils are pure and unadulterated.

This advice is especially important for the Professional Aromatherapist if buying oils outside the normal sphere of the profession.

Professional Aromatherapists will not usually be in the position of having to buy oils 'over the counter' where perhaps temperature and storage might not be ideal.

A HISTORY OF AROMATHERAPY
THROUGH THE AGES

The first step in the history of Aromatherapy is probably almost as old as man himself. It is impossible to date when flowers, plants and roots were first used for medicinal purposes.

Early man discovered that some of the branches and twigs that he burned on his fire for warmth caused changes in mood; some giving feelings of wellbeing, some giving feelings of drowsiness. Inevitably it was realised that the aromas of the smoke helped with difficult breathing and congestion.

Early man depended on Nature's larder of fruits, berries, roots and leaves not only for the food he ate but to cure the sick and heal his wounds. It is also feasible that he gained some of his knowledge of the benefits of plants by studying sick animals to see what they ate and how they reacted. As the reason behind the healing properties of plants was unknown the communities tended to attribute the process to a God or Gods. Styrax was linked with Saturn, Costus with Mars, Myrrh with the Moon, and Incense with the Sun. Osiers was the God of Vegetation and his twin sister had the power to renew life.

THE EGYPTIANS

To the ancient Egyptians medicine was a way of life. They are known to have used Myrrh, Frankincense, Cedarwood, Origanum, Bitter Almond, Spikenard, Henna, Juniper, Coriander and Calamus. Their love of flowers is depicted in many of their earliest wall paintings.

Various medical papyrus dating back to 2000 BC have been discovered by archaeologists in the last 100 years. These list a number of recipes in use after 1800 BC, the majority being of vegetable base. Each recipe described the condition as well as its symptoms and gave clear instructions on how the medication should be prepared and administered.

Plants and herbs were used not only for medicinal purposes but also for embalming the dead. This showed great knowledge of plants and herbs as well as of anatomy.

Cedarwood was one of the oils used in mummification. Its use can be attributed to the fact that it was considered to be imperishable. Several centuries later the mummified bodies found in the tombs were well preserved and this has been attributed to the antibacterial and antiseptic properties of the oils.

The Egyptians used infused oils. They also used a form of enfleurage to extract their oils. It is quite possible to assume from some of the findings and records that the Egyptians practised a method of distillation. Should this prove to be true, distillation would have been known to the Egyptians at least 2000 years before the Arabians were supposed to have invented the process.

The Egyptians treated hayfever with a mixture of antimony, aloes, myrrh and honey and went on to discover a spermicide which was a blend of acacia coloquinte, dates and honey.

Kyphi or Khypi, the oldest form of perfume known to man, (a mixture of sixteen different oils), was very popular with the Egyptians both in the home and for use by the priests in the temples. When archeologists opened the tomb of Tutankhamun (reign 1361-1352 BC) in 1922 the smell of Kyphi was said to have emanated from it. The archeologists found scent pots and vases, some contained ungents (an ointment). Although the scent was faint it was still detectable and later it was possible to establish the identity of some of the contents of the pots. The tomb had been sealed in 1350 BC, during the reign of Khufa who built the great Pyramid.

Earlier still when the tomb of King Menes (3000 BC) was opened in 1897 it was found to have the remains of aromatic products present.

In 1978 archaeologists divulged the secrets of Queen Nefertiti's beauty. It is said that she used beauty cleansing masks of honey, milk and flower pollens. To keep her skin soft she also bathed in a bath containing oils from eighty different fruits and herbs as well as using a lotion of honey and orchid leaves. The last Queen of Egypt, Cleopatra, is said to have seduced Mark Antony by her lavish use of perfume.

When Egypt collapsed all knowledge of deciphering the Hieroglyphics disappeared. The Rosetta Stone in the British Museum holds the key to the Hieroglyphics and this dates from the time of Ptolemy V (Macedonian king of Egypt 205 BC). The same passage is written three times in three different languages, Demotic, Hieroglyphics and Greek. As we can understand Greek it has therefore been possible to decipher the other two languages.

MESOPOTAMIA

Mesopotamia (modern Iraq) has a history going back to the Akkadians, Assyrians, Babylonians and the Sumarians whom it is believed were the first people to develop writing. The region is one of the earliest centres of civilised life.

The Babylonian doctors recorded their prescriptions on clay tablets and gave clear details as to when and how a remedy should be prepared and taken. What they did not record however, was the quantities to be used.

Like the Egyptians the Summarians believed that sickness was the manifestation of devils and evil spirits. What we do not know is who influenced whom in this belief.

Kings of the day established gardens of medicinal plants. Many of these plants are still in use today; they include : Apricot, Myrrh, Poppy, Sesame, Garlic, Onion, Fennel, Rose and Juniper.

ANCIENT GREECE

This ancient civilization took much from the Egyptian and Mesopotamian worlds including their knowledge of medicine. This gave the Greeks great stepping stones for advancement in making further discoveries as well as laying the foundations for a scientific basis to medicine.

They used perfumed oils for cosmetic and medicinal purposes. Soldiers were given ointment of Myrrh to carry with them to help heal the wounds of war.

Marestheus a Greek physician, recognised that aromatic plants and flowers had either stimulating or sedative properties.

Theophrastus - Father of Botany, recommended the use of olive oil to absorb the perfume of the aromatic oil as this prolonged the life of the scent.

Hippocrates - Father of Medicine (460-377 BC) was the first person known to establish and set down a scientific system of medicine, a system of diagnosis and prognosis. He used over 400 drugs of vegetable origin in his prescriptions and studies.

Two of Hippocrates most famous quotations are:

"There is a cure on earth for every ill".
and
"A wise man ought to realise that health is his most valuable possession and learn how to treat illnesses by his own judgement".

Many famous Greeks worked for the Romans.
Galen - Born 13AD in Turkey (which was then under Greek rule), was physician to Marcus Aurelius and was the first physician to discover the pulse; he is also credited with the original Cold Cream. An outstanding writer, Galen recorded a great deal on the theory of plant medicine and plant classification.

Dioscorides - The chief physician to Nero, had by 78 AD collected information on plants from all around the Mediterranean.

He left us his recordings in "Materia Medica" which contained information not only on the plants but also their uses. For example, he praised the onion for its diuretic and tonic properties and its effectiveness against infection.

Centuries later his theories about the onion were proved in that its juices worked as an antibiotic against staphylococcus and other microbes. Onion has also been used by the Australian aborigines to ward off infection.

Pliny - His encyclopedia of 37 volumes had no less than 16 volumes devoted to plants. His works represented the writings and findings of almost 400 different authors and although they contained much misinformation they also contained a lot of information that would otherwise have been unavailable to us, as many of the previous studies to which he referred have been destroyed.

The fall of the Roman Empire around 400AD caused Roman physicians to flee to Constantinople; from here their knowledge was passed to the Arabs.

THE ARABIANS

Although it is customary to speak of Arabian medicine in this period not all physicians of the day were Arabs or natives. Neither were they all Muslims, some were Jews and some Christians. They were drawn from all areas of the empire stretching along the entire coast of Africa and into Spain. They were great traders and spread their knowledge throughout the world of the day. The Arabs discovered alcohol, which meant that perfumes could be made without a heavy oil base.

Aly-Ali-Ibn-Sina, more commonly known as Avicenna (980-1037 AD), is considered to have been one of the greatest Arab physicians. Some say that if Hippocrates is thought of as the Father of Medicine then surely Avicenna could be considered, amongst other things to be the Father of Massage and Manipulation. He laid down clear guidelines for massage and originated various forms of manipulations for spinal problems as well as inventing the idea of traction for broken limbs. He was an outstanding scholar, being an accepted doctor by the age of eighteen years. At twenty one he was famed for his mastery of formal learning and medical prowess.

He built on the works of Hippocrates, Galen and Dioscorides whose recordings were translated into Persian and other Arab languages. In his own works Avicenna described eight hundred plants and their uses.

In spite of his many achievements, including being made Physician in Chief to a hospital in Bagdad, he was to spend long periods in prison, brought about by the jealousy and intrigue of others. Avicennas's two most famed works were the Book of Healing and Canon of Medicine. He is also credited with having perfected and by some accredited with the invention of distillation.

EUROPEANS IN GENERAL AND THE MIDDLE AGES

ELEVENTH CENTURY

No real recordings exist between the Eleventh and Twelfth Century; a period known as The Dark Ages.

TWELFTH CENTURY

Knights in the Crusades brought back knowledge of perfumes and how to distil oils. The perfumers of Arabia were now famous throughout Europe. Recipes were available and due to the advent of printing, books called Herbals were published, giving information on plants and prescriptions.

THIRTEENTH CENTURY

The development of distillation was now being encouraged by the new pharmaceutical industry. Not having the same plants as the Orientals the Europeans adapted quickly, using native shrubs and plants; Rosemary, Lavender and Thyme being amongst the many.
The distillation coincided with the achievements of the famous Bologna School of Medicine, which incidentally is credited with having contributed greatly to anaesthesia. Their prescription for anaesthetic was to soak into a sponge the juices of plants which had been previously boiled and stored for use.

It is now generally accepted that this method of anaesthetic originated in India many years before. During this period St. Hildegarde, the Abbess of Bingen, wrote four theses on medicinal plants. Her works are still referred to today.

THE RENAISSANCE

FOURTEENTH CENTURY

In the fourteenth century (1340-1350) the first plague hit Europe. Known as The Black Death, it killed almost half of Europe's population. The only protection available against disease, at that time, was the use of aromatic plant material, e.g. herbs, plants and flowers. These were strewn onto the floors, burned in the streets and carried on the person in public in the form of pomanders.

FIFTEENTH CENTURY

Gildemeister's writings informs us that the oils of Bitter Almond, Cedar, Cinnamon, Frankincense, Mastic, Rose and Sage were well known. During the next two years sixty more essential oils were added to the list. J.M. Feminis created the first Eau Admirable which was further developed by his nephew and is known today as Eau de Cologne (a proven antiseptic).
The practice of covering the floor with aromatic plants continued, as did the use of pomanders and lavender bags to ward off disease. In 1492 Columbus landed in the Bahamas. From then on the explorers brought back many herbs, spices and plants.

SIXTEENTH AND SEVENTEENTH CENTURIES

Throughout the middle ages and Tudor times all forms of plant medicine were used by apothecaries, doctors and lay people. This period saw the flourishing growth of the perfumery industry and the periods are noted as the great herbal times of Europe.

The now well established and practised art of herb-strewing on the floors continued to be enacted to create pleasant smells and help prevent the spread of disease. The gentlemen of the day, including the medical practitioners, carried a little cassolette filled with aromatics on the top of their walking sticks. This was raised to the nose in the presence of disease or foul smells; it was considered a personal antiseptic. The 17th century has been referred to as the 'Golden Age of Herbalists' such as Nicholas Culpepper, John Parkinson, John Gerard in England; Otto Brunfels, Leonard Fuchs and Hieronymus Boch in Germany; Nicholas Monasdes in Spain; Pietro Mattioli in Italy and Charles de L'Ecluse in France.

Culpepper (born 1616) tried to make medicine available to all people and gave treatment free to the poor. He published the English Physician (now known as Culpepper's Herbal) in 1653; it contained 369 medicines made of English herbs.

It is believed that Culpepper gained a lot of his knowledge from the writings of Galen.

Mattioli's herbal was translated into a number of European languages and sold 32,000 copies. His work was based on the writings of Dioscorides.

Essential oils were being used not only by herbalists but also by doctors; a trend which continued until the end of the 19th century.

From 1665 to the Great Fire in 1666 there raged the second outbreak of plague. The disease was dealt with in a similar way to that of three hundred years before; it had been noted that the perfumers and those wearing perfumed gloves remained almost immune to the diseases of the time.

One outcome from this tragic time was a growing new science of experimental chemistry; the forerunner to the use of chemical substances in medicine.

THE FAR EAST, INDIA AND CHINA

No earlier civilisations exist. These two civilisations survived and have a continuing history today. Both grew up around major rivers. In India the Ganges and in China the Huang (yellow).

The use of plants for healing has an unbroken record for thousands of years, unlike Europe, where we are now only beginning to rediscover our broken heritage of knowledge.

INDIA

In India the oldest form of medicine is Ayurveda. Ayur meaning Life and Veda meaning Knowledge. No synthetic material is used in this medicine. Ayurvedic is mainly plant based, although some animal and mineral material is used. In Ayurveda it is believed that our direct link to the universe which surrounds us is through our senses. To feel, to hear, to see, to smell and to taste is to perceive. In India the Lotus flower grows in abundance along the lakes in Kashmir, where the flower is the symbol of rejuvenation.

Lord Shiva, one of the Gods of the Hindu faith is referred to as "The First Herbalist".

Asoka, emperor of India in 3 BC, is said to have established eighteen institutions with some characteristics similar to those of modern hospitals, in that cleanliness was stressed and diet therapy as well as treatment with herbs, plants and oils was practised; but above all patients were treated with kindness.

He organised and regulated the cultivation of medicinal plants. Great attention was paid to the conditions in which the plants grew and to those who tended them. The medicinal plants of India form the basis of present day traditional medicine in that country.

The Indians' ancient language is Sanskrit, which was written on Olapalm leaves. They were dried out and cut into strips and strung together to make a book. The leaves had a strong durability which prevented them from crumbling.

CHINA

Like India, China has an unbroken tradition of herbal medicine. The earliest known records are in the "Yellow Emperors' Classics of Internal Medicine" dating back to 2000 BC. It deals mainly with causes and treatment of disease. Another great classic of Chinese herbal medicine known as Pen-Tsao- Khang-Mou, lists 816 different formulae taken from almost 20,000 different substances, most being of plant origin.

The Chinese used opium as a treatment for dysentery from as early as 1000 BC but did not begin to smoke opium until the Ming Dynasty in the sixteenth century when alcohol was banned. The Chinese written language is composed of ideograms, ideas strung together with characters. The original materials were lacquer on bamboo. The bamboo was cut into strips and the people wrote from top to bottom due to the shape of the bamboo and the strips were then strung together to make books. Ancient Chinese books look like curtains.

THE 18TH AND 19TH CENTURIES

During the 18th and 19th centuries chemists continued to research the active ingredients of medicinal plants and identified a number of substances (some narcotics) including quinine and morphine. During this period a fairly familiar substance of our present day was also discovered, 'caffeine'.

Although in this new era chemists/scientists were able to investigate and research more plants in a real scientific way the tendency was growing to isolate the active principals of plants. This led to the replacement of the use of a great number of essential oils by synthetic substances and many have indeed been very effective but against the success has to be measured the side effects of some.

THE 20th CENTURY

Essential oils continued to be used by the pharmaceutical industry into the present century. Until the 20th century essential oils had been classified along with herbal remedies and cosmetics.

Our modern knowledge of Aromatherapy stems from the early 1920's. Although progress with research and discoveries was slow and somewhat random. William Minchin, the English doctor, discovered the benefits of Garlic oil and had great success in treating patients with T.B. and diphtheria. The Italian doctors Giovanni Gatti and Renato Cayola were working on the psychotherapeutic applications of essential oils. The Australian doctor Penfold was working with Tea-Tree oil. Research was also taking place in the USA, Japan and the former USSR.

It was a french cosmetic chemist, Renée Gattefosse who coined the term 'Aromatherapie' in 1937. Gattefosse is looked on as the father of Aromatherapy; his interests were in the antimicrobial effects of the oils and in their application to the skin for both cosmetic and medicinal purposes. He published both a scientific paper and book. His personal interest in the use of Lavender oil for the treatment of burns was aroused following an accident in the laboratory in which he badly burned his hand. To ease the pain he put his hand into the nearest bowl of essential oil; this happened to be Lavender. The burn healed quickly leaving no trace of a scar. He continued his research into essential oils publishing a book entitled 'Aromatherapy'.

The progress of Aromatherapy came almost to a standstill with the Second World War. The notable exception being doctor Jean Valnet. He had been influenced by the work of Gattefosse and was using essential oils as antiseptics when treating soldiers. After the war he continued to use the oils; he also taught other doctors how to use the oils. Today there are numerous doctors in France using essential oils and many fine training establishments where medical doctors can learn the art.

France was to give the next great Aromatherapist of our time a chance to explore and work with the oils in a much wider field. Marguerite Maury, born in Austria, had a great love for botany and biochemistry. She married at a very early age and after a number of tragic incidents in her life she qualified as a nurse and surgical assistant. She moved to France where she worked for many years as a nursing assistant to a surgeon in Alsace. It was while there that she was given a book which had been written by Dr. Chabenes, published in 1838 (the author later taught Dr. Gattefosse). The book became Marguerite's bible. She dedicated her life to Aromatherapy and tried to prove the value of essential oil on the wellbeing of people. She lectured and gave seminars on the subject in France, Switzerland and England. Marguerite Maury ran courses for and lectured to Beauty Therapists, who during the sixties became the first Aromatherapists in England. I was one of those lucky therapists.

After just one or two years the practice of including Aromatherapy as part of the training in Beauty Therapy stopped. It became no longer necessary for the Beauty Therapist to learn about the individual oils he/she could purchase and use. The Beauty Therapist began to use pre-blended oils in massage; this is a practice which continues in some training in the UK and other countries today and has led to confusion amongst members of the public.

Today Aromatherapy is used in most walks of life and practised within the health service of many countries.

BASIC BIOLOGY OF PLANTS AND FLOWERS

Plants and animals, including man, owe their existence to the presence of a complicated chemical substance known as Deoxyribonucleic Acid or DNA for short. This material contains the genes and controls the activities of the organism.

Life is literally dependent on the presence of this DNA. Plants are similar to man in other ways; not least in that there are substantial areas of function that are not completely understood.

The basic units from which plants develop are called cells. These exist in a wide variety of shapes and forms, each type specialised to carry out a particular function. Each cell's length, width and thickness is regulated by chemical reaction.

The growth of a whole plant involves the growth of roots, stems, leaves, flowers and other structures. For a healthy plant to grow there has to be a continuous supply of new cells to add to those already in existence. The supply of these new cells is achieved by a process of cell division. In the later life of the plant, when the roots and stems begin to thicken (a process known as secondary thickening), there is further cell division.

THE ROOT OF THE PLANT

The root of the plant performs two important functions in the life of the plant.

1. It provides firm support for the rest of the plant by anchoring these roots firmly to the ground.

2. The roots extract water and dissolved nutrients from the soil.

STEMS

The main functions of the stem are:-

1. To provide support for the leaves and flowers in such a way as they can best absorb sunlight.

2. To provide a transport system for the distribution of substances within the plant.

LEAVES

The function of a leaf is almost always the same whatever the shape. That function is the production of energy. The cells of a leaf contain pigment (a coloured substance), the most important being chlorophyll which absorbs light from the sun's rays. This is converted into a form of energy and this energy is then used to power a series of reactions, a process which is known as Photosynthesis (because it depends on light).

During this process plants take in carbon dioxide directly from the air. It enters the leaf through minute pores called stoma found on the surface of the leaf. Oxygen is a by-product of photosynthesis. Put simply, molecules of water are split into the two elements, hydrogen and oxygen, of which they are composed. Some of the oxygen is used by the plant, the remainder is released into the air. The hydrogen combines with the carbon from carbon-dioxide to form various kinds of plant sugars which are called carbohydrates. Without photosynthesis the human race could not survive as there would be nothing to eat. This must surely make photosynthesis one of the most important processes on earth.

FLOWERS

Flowers are believed by most people to be the most beautiful and interesting part of a plant. Flowers are arranged in spirals or whorls around a central stalk. Flowers consist of four component parts:-

1 . Sepals
They look like tiny leaves and are collectively known as calyx. Their function is mainly protective.

2. Petals
These are found just inside the sepals. In some flowers the sepals and the flowers are not very distinct. The petals are normally brightly coloured in order to attract insects, which is important for the process of pollination and the life cycle of the plant.

3. Stamen
This is the male reproductive part of the flower arranged around the centre of the flower. The stamen consists of a slender stalk called a filament which ends in saclike structures called Anthers. It is inside the anthers that thousands of pollen grains are produced. These pollen grains contain the male sex cell or gamete, which can fertilise a female egg cell.

4. Pistil
This is the female reproductive part of the plant found in the centre of the flower. The pistil consists of a protective structure called the Ovary or Carpel. This contains one or more ovules and one or more female egg cell is contained in each ovule. At the top of the ovary is a slender projection called the style; this ends in a specialised pollen receiving region known as the stigma.   For fertilisation to take place the male sex cell (a pollen grain) must become attached to the stigma.   It then germinates to produce a pollen tube which grows through the style to reach the ovule.   The male and female sex cells fuse and an embryo is formed which may grow into a new plant.

Note!
Not all plants contain both the male and female reproductive parts.

POLLINATION

In self-pollination plant grains are transported from the anthers to stigma on the same individual plant, whereas in cross pollination plant pollen is transferred to the stigmas of different individuals of the same species.

INFLORESCENCE

The way flowers can be grouped together in arrangements is called inflorescence and this can be important in identifying flowers.

Some of the common types of inflorescence are:-

Spike, Raceme, Panicle, Cyme, Umbel, Capitulum.

PLANT MATERIAL

There are various systems for classifying plant material. The most common is the Organographic System. This classifies the plant's raw material according to the part of the plant gathered.

Subterranean refers to the part of the plant that is located below the ground. These parts are as follows :-

COMMON NAME	TECHNICAL NAME
Bulb	Bulbus
Rhizome	Rhizoma
Root	Radix
Tuber	Tuber

The parts of the plant visible above the ground are as follows :-

COMMON NAME	TECHNICAL NAME
Bark	Cortex
Bud	Gemma
Fruit	Fructus
Flower	Flos
Glands	Glandulae
Herb	Herba
Leaf	Folium
Seed	Semen
Stalk	Caulis
Stipe	Stipe

CLASSIFICATION OF PLANTS

Through his books Genera Plantarum and Critica Botanica published in 1737 the great Swedish botanist Carl Von Linné, usually known as Carl Linnaeus, formalised a new scientific language - Botanical Latin. In this language each species was given a two part Latin name (binomial). This name was unique and separated the name and description.

The first part of the Latin name denotes the genus and may be shared by many other species. The second part either commemorates a famous botanist (often the person who discovered it) or refers to some feature of the species.

Linnaeus based his botanical classification on the number of carpels and stamens. This was an artificial system which led to some anomalies. Through time and in the light of new knowledge small parts of his original works were revised, though most of the genera he classified still remains the same. A great number of botanical names are still followed by the suffix 'L'. A tribute to his accuracy.

In spite of the general acceptance internationally of the rules of nomenclature, plants have been named and described by a number of different people which can still sometimes cause confusion.

Although we use 21 plant families and approximately 240 plants in Aromatherapy to obtain essential oils just 16 families produce the most well-known and respected essential oils.

PLANT FAMILIES

ANNONANCEAE

Over 2,000 species make up this almost entirely tropical family of trees and shrubs. In the tropics various species are used for medicine, ointment and perfume.

OILS OF THIS FAMILY:

Ylang-Ylang   - Canarga Odorata

BURSERACEAE

A plant of the desert and tropics credited with anti-inflammatory powers.

OILS OF THIS FAMILY:

Frankincense   - Boswellia Carterii
Myrrh   - Commiphora Myrrha

COMPOSITAE

The largest botanical family, these plants grow mainly in open spaces in most parts of the world. The exceptions being the tropical forests and the most northerly regions. Credited with a great diversity of healing powers.

OILS OF THIS FAMILY:

Chamomile German   - Matricaria Chamomilla
Chamomile Roman   - Anthemis Nobilis

CUPRESSACEAE

The name Conifer implies a tree that bears cones and needles. Conifers are amongst the oldest and highest trees in the world and are found in both Northern and Southern hemispheres. From this family come many producers of paper and wood pulp as well as essential oils.

OILS OF THIS FAMILY:

Juniper	- Juniperus Communis
Cypress	- Cupressus Sempervirens
Cedarwood	- Cedrus Atlantica

GERANIACEAE

The plant of strong adaptability. Geranium Robertianum is the wild geranium found in various parts of the temperate world. It is totally different to the types used for the extraction of oils; namely Pelargonium Graveolens and Pelargonium Odrantissimum (rose scented).

OILS OF THIS FAMILY:

Geranium	- Pelargonium Graveolens
	- Pelargonium Odorantissimum

GRAMINEAE

The nutritious plants of the earth; its intricate network of roots blending with the soil. Graminae include not only the common grasses but also barley, corn, oats, rice and wheat as well as the tropical spices.

OILS OF THIS FAMILY:

Lemongrass	- Cymbopogan Citratus
Palma Rosa	- Cymbopogon Martinii

LABIATAE

The plants associated with curative powers. They are found in open spaces in moderate climates and tend to be those that we think of in culinary terms as herbs.

OILS OF THE FAMILY:

Basil	- Ocimum Basilicum
Clary-Sage	- Salvia Sclarea
Lavender	- Lavandula Officinalis
Marjoram	- Origamun Marjorana
Melissa	- Melissa Officinalis
Patchouli	- Pogostemon Cablin
	- Pogostemon Patchouli
Peppermint	- Mentha Piperita
Rosemary	- Rosmarinus
Thyme	- Thymus Vulgaris

LAURACEAE

About 2,500 species make up this family of trees and shrubs. They are almost exclusively tropical and are all extremely aromatic.

OILS OF THE FAMILY:

Cinnamon Leaf - Cinnamomum Zeylanicum

MYRTACEAE

The plant of harmony. It grows mainly in the tropics.

OILS OF THE FAMILY:

Cajuput	- Melaleuca Leucodendron
	- Melaleuca Cajeputi
Eucalyptus	- Eucalyptus Globulus
Niaouli	- Melaleuca Viridiflora
Tea-Tree	- Melaleuca Alternifolia

OLEACEAE

Shrubs and tree of the sub tropical or temperate climates. The name Jasmine is derived from the Persian Yasmin. It belongs to the genus Jasminum from the family Oleaceae.

OILS OF THIS FAMILY:

Jasmine	- Grandiflorum	Essential Oil
Jasmine	- Officinale	Essential oil
Jasmine	- Sambac	Scenting Tea
Jasmine	- Panticulatum	(China) Scenting Tea

PINACEAE

The Scots Pine is the only pine native to Great Britain and its range extends through Europe, Asia and the former USSR. There are numerous different forms varying in colour, needles, size, shape and cones.

OILS OF THIS FAMILY:

Pine	- Pinus Sylverstris

PIPERACEAE

About 1,000 species into 10 genera. Distributed throughout the tropics. Used in medicine, food and beverages.

OILS OF THIS FAMILY:

Black Pepper - Piper Nigrum

RUTACEAE

Plants/trees of this Rue family number more than 1,600 grouped into about 150 genera. They are found in tropical, subtropical and temperate regions.
The oils produced by this family are refreshing and cooling. It has been known for some handlers of the essential oils from the Rutaceae family to develop dermatitis.

OILS OF THIS FAMILY:

Bergamot	- Citrus Bergamia
Mandarin	- Citrus Madurensis
Grapefruit	- Citrus Paradisi
Neroli	- Citrus Aurantium
	- Citrus Vulgaris
Lemon	- Citrus Paradisi
Lime	- Citrus Aurantifolia
Petitgrain	- Citrus Aurantum
Tangerine	- Citrus Reticulata
Violet	- Viola Odorata

ROSACEAE

3000 or more species in 100 genera of the Rose family.

OILS OF THIS FAMILY:

Rose   - Rose Centifolia
                      - Rosa Damascena

SANTALACEAE

The Sandalwood family of shrubs and trees; all of semiparasitic nature and consisting of some 400 species grouped into 30 genera. This family is found in tropical and temperate regions.

OILS OF THIS FAMILY:

Sandalwood   - Santalum Album

STYRACEAE

About 175 species of trees and shrubs grouped into twelve genera widely distributed. Some species produce aromatic resins.

OILS OF THIS FAMILY:

Benzoin   - Styrax Benzoin

UMBELLIFERAE

A family of 3,000 species in about 300 genera. Found mainly in the temperate zones of the northern hemisphere with a considerable number occurring wild in the USA.

OILS OF THIS FAMILY:

Fennel Sweet   - Foeniculum Vulgare

VIOLACEAE

More than 900 species found all over the world but not the arctic. The European Violet is the most sweetly scented.

OILS OF THIS FAMILY:

Violet   - Viola Odorata

ZINGIBERACEAE

Ginger (Zingiber Officinale) is noted for its medicinal properties and has been used for thousands of years in China and India.

OILS OF THIS FAMILY:

Ginger   - Zingiber Officinale

HOW ARE THE OILS EXTRACTED FROM THE PLANTS?

Essential oil is produced by a variety of methods.

DISTILLATION

The most common method used to obtain the oils is steam distillation. In this method the plant is held in a container above boiling water. The steam produced by the water draws off the essential oil. The oil and steam travel to a further collecting chamber where the steam is cooled to form water in which the essential oil will either sink to the bottom or float to the top depending on its density. The water is then drawn off leaving only the essential oil.

ENFLEURAGE

The procedure for obtaining essential oil by the enfleurage method is extremely labour intensive and no longer widely used.

Chassis, the name given to the wooden framed glass (much like small windows in appearance) are prepared by coating the glass with a film of specially purified fat. Freshly picked flowers are placed on to the layers of fat and the chassis are then stacked one above the other. After some time (between 24 and 70 hours) the wilted flowers are removed and more fresh flowers are added to the enfleurage.

The enfleurage (fat mixture) becomes saturated with essential oil and is now called pomade (this product can be used as an ointment or perfume).

The pomade is then mixed with alcohol. The essential oil dissolves but the fat is insoluble in the alcohol and is drained off. The next step is to gently heat the alcohol so that it evaporates, leaving the essential oil in the container.

EUCELLE

This was a traditional method of obtaining the oils from the citrus family (particularly lemons). Revolving barrel-type drums lined with spikes were packed with citrus fruits. The movement jarred the fruit against the spikes, puncturing it and releasing the oil to be drained off and stored.

EXPRESSION

This method is reserved for citrus fruits. The rind is grated or squeezed into a sponge and when the sponge becomes saturated the oil is squeezed into a container. Since the 1930's machines have taken over from man for this process. The workers involved in handling the sponges full of essential oils used to suffer quite severe allergic reactions especially on the hands. Hence this is one area where the machine is welcomed to take over the job of man.

MACERATION

This is a similar method to enfleurage. The part of the plant to be used is plunged into hot fat which penetrates the cells of the plant, absorbing their oils. When the fat is saturated the process to collect the essential oil is then performed. This process is the same as that performed in the second stage of enfleurage. It should be noted that in this method the plant is sometimes crushed or broken up prior to or during the process of obtaining the oil.

SOLVENT

Solvent extraction is a complicated process. The flowers, gums or resins are placed in a container and covered with a solvent to extract the oil. This is followed by various heating, cooling and filtering processes which result in a dark coloured paste known as a Concrete. To obtain an absolute from the concrete alcohol is added into which a number of the constituents dissolve. The alcohol is then evaporated off completely and the resulting mix is known as an Absolute. In order to obtain an essential oil free from nonvolatile residual wax the absolutes can be subjected to a further method of processing known as molecular distillation.

HYPERCRITICAL CARBON DIOXIDE EXTRACTION

Hypercritical carbon dioxide extraction is one of the later methods used for obtaining essential oil from the plant; it is one of the quickest methods and yet one of the most expensive. The latter is due in part to the cost of building the very expensive heavy stainless steel equipment necessary to cope with the high pressures (200 times higher than regular atmospheric pressure). This method of extraction takes place in a closed chamber at a fairly low temperature. Therefore the fragrance is not affected by heat and even the most volatile and fragile fraction of the fragrance can be collected, leaving the end product very close to the plant's aromatic substance. The extraction method takes but a few minutes in comparison to between 1 and 48 hours for steam distillation.

Why Carbon Dioxide ? The benefit of extraction is threefold - low temperature, speed and quality of return. Any substance can exist in three different states - gas, liquid and solid. Each substance may be in anyone of these three states depending on its temperature and pressure. In addition to this certain substances can be found in the hypercritical state, that is they are neither gas nor liquid but rather they are both; they have solvent properties and can disperse as readily as a gas, i.e. almost instantaneously. Carbon dioxide, a gas naturally occurring in the air we breath, has the power to become hypercritical. As its hypercritical temperature is only 33°C it is an excellent solvent for use in obtaining Aromatherapy oils.

DEFINITION OF SOME TERMS USED IN EXTRACTION/OBTAINING ESSENTIAL OILS

Absolutes:
Aromatic material extracted from the plant using solvent extraction. The extract is more viscous (sticky) than essential oil and tends to be quite coloured. Absolutes may contain some residual amounts of solvent.

Concrete:
A dark coloured paste which contains natural waxes, odoriferous molecules and some chemical residue (the result of solvent extraction prior to the addition of pure alcohol).

Pomades:
Pomades are the oil laden fat products of a process known as Enfleurage.

Resinoid:
The result of solvent extraction on dead organic matter e.g. Benzoin, Frankincense, Myrrh. Further distillation will yield an essential oil of Myrrh and Frankincense but not of Benzoin as its aromatic constituents are insufficiently volatile.

Note !
Gums are soluble in water and not in alcohol.
Resins are soluble in alcohol and not in water.

Adulteration:
Can be taken to mean any changes made to the pure essential oil.

Biocides :
Herbicides and pesticides are known collectively as Biocides and traces of biocides can be found in essential oils, whether the oil is expressed or distilled. Absolutes are even more likely to retain biocides.

Contaminants:
May include pesticides and this could feasibly increase the potential toxicity.

Cutting:
Mixing an original oil to make it go further using a number of alternatives.

Degradation:
Lessening of the essential oil's properties caused by three main factors - atmospheric oxygen, heat and light. These changes are not usually intentional and certainly not desirable in essential oils.

Dilution:
Using chemicals or fixed oils to make the essential oil go further (increase volume).

Fabrication:
A combination of the components that would be found naturally in a specific oil but contains none of the named specific oil, e.g. Melissa Oil - the majority of the oil on the market is of this type.

Note!
Could be considered as made up by man using Nature's supplies to copy from.

Folding:
Batches of the same oil mixed and stored for up to two years followed by further processing, e.g. deterpination of terpenes or sesquiterpenes.

Nature Identical:
Essential oil composed of components obtained from plant sources which may or may not be from the same species of plant.

Oxidation:
The addition of oxygen or the removal of electrons or hydrogen from an organic molecule which changes the efficacy of an essential oil and may render the oil more hazardous due to chemical change. Some changes may lead to an oil becoming a skin sensitizer.

Rectification:
Can encompass a number of changes and is often referred to as adulteration. In its true sense rectification suggests removing a component from the oil, e.g. deterpination (removal of terpenes from citrus oils to prolong shelf life).

Substitutions:
Normally means using a cheaper essential oil e.g. Petitgrain for Neroli.

Synthetics:
Composed of chemical components made in laboratory from various starting materials (it is often difficult for the average person to distinguish between them and the real thing).

CHEMICAL CONSTITUENTS OF ESSENTIAL OILS

The chemical constituents of essential oils are determined by two factors:

1. Intrinsic factors (occurring within the plant)

These are the internal processes in the plant cells that make each individual type of plant produce a different range of end products from simple hydrogen and carbon building blocks. The way in which the building blocks are able to combine in different permutations is determined by the genetic make up of each plant type.

2. Extrinsic factors (occurring outside the plant)

Many factors can introduce subtle changes in the combination of individual constituents. The growing conditions of the plant, e.g. soil type, climate and harvesting processes should be considered. By far the greatest factor is the extraction process by which the oil is obtained. The action of heat and steam in the distillation process creates chemicals in the essential oils that are not present naturally in the living plants.

One important fact which should be remembered by all therapists is that one of the special characteristics of essential oil molecules is their size is very small; this is one fact that is credited (by some) with enabling the essential oil to penetrate the skin.

CLASSIFICATIONS OF CONSTITUENTS

From a therapeutic point of view the following classifications of constituents of essential oils may be found to be most useful :

TERPENES (SUFFIXED - ENE)

Terpenes are hydrocarbons consisting of hydrogen and carbon atoms. They are unsaturated molecules, (i.e. contain one or more carbon atoms double bond) which allows them to react easily with oxygen to produce the terpenoids. Three classes of terpenes are found in essential oils.

MONOTERPENES (MONOCYCLIC/ BICYCLIC)

These have a 10 carbon atom backbone. They are small enough to distil with steam and are the main constituents of many essential oils. Monoterpenes such as Limonene and Pinene have antiviral and antiseptic properties respectively.

SESQUITERPENES

These have a 15 atom backbone and are also commonly found molecules in essential oils. In spite of being less volatile than the monoterpenes they can still be distilled with steam. Essential oils with a high proportion of sesquiterpene constituents are mostly distilled from roots and woods or from plants of the Compositae family. Chamomile oil contains Chamazulene and the sesquiterpenoid Farnesol, both of which have anti-inflammatory and antibacterial properties.

DITERPENES

These have 20 carbon atoms, are less common in essential oils and not readily steam distilled.

OXYGENATED DERIVATIVES

The most common are oxygen derivatives of terpenes

ALDEHYDES - (SUFFIXED - AL or ALDEHYDE)

The monoterpenoid aldehydes Citral and Citronellal are the principal chemical features of such oils as Melissa and Citronella. Many examples have sedative and/or antiseptic properties. Structurally the oxygen is attached to a carbon linked to a hydrogen and the functional group is located at the end of a carbonic chain.

KETONES - (SUFFIXED - ONE)

This functional group is produced by the attachment of an oxygen atom to a carbon atom within the carbonic chain. Ketones are among the most toxic constituents found in essential oils. They are found in Wormwood, Sage, Tansy, Pulegone, and Pennyroyal. Not all ketones are toxic and the therapist needs to look at them carefully.

ESTERS - (SUFFIXED - ATE)

The ester functional group contains 2 oxygen atoms. The second oxygen atom is bonded to the carbon of the carboxyl group. Esters are produced through the reaction of an alcohol with an acid, i.e. Linalol + Acetic acid = Linalyl Acetate (principal ester in Lavender, Clary Sage) + Water. Esters are among the most widespread group found in essential oils and have both sedative and fungicidal properties. They provide the finer notes to many fragrances.

ALCOHOLS (SUFFIXED - OL or ALCOHOL)

Oxygen is attached to the carbon atom of the parent molecule through a single bond in the hydroxyl group in which hydrogen takes up the second bond. These are among the most useful group of compounds. They are generally non-toxic and are uplifting with antiviral and antiseptic qualities.

PHENOLS - (ALSO SUFFIXED - OL)

Structurally in this group, the hydroxyl group is attached to a benzene ring. Thymol and Carvacrol, found in Thyme, are very strong antibacterials and in common with other phenols have strong stimulating effects. They should be used only in appropriately low concentrations as they can cause skin irritation.

OXIDES

The most important oxide is Eucalyptol (Cineole) which is the principal constituent of Eucalyptus oil. It is found to a lesser degree in Rosemary, Tea-Tree and Cajuput and has a strong expectorant effect.

PHENYLPROPANES

These compounds have a phenyl ring system with a propane (three carbon atom) side chain. This (nine carbon atom) structure can be modified by various functional groups added to it, as in the terpenes. The special electron configuration in these structures allows some pharmacologically highly active molecules to be produced. Like the phenols Cinnamic Aldehyde and Eugenol (found in Cinnamon and Clove respectively), they are very strong antiseptics but used in excess can cause severe skin reactions. Other examples such as Methyl Chavicol and Myristicin (Nutmeg) can cause negative effects if used in unreasonably high concentrations.

Other molecules occur in plants but do not find their way to the essential oil. The reason for their absence is that their molecule size or weight is too high to evaporate with steam.

NOTE !
The suffixes quoted above are only a guide to the constituents group, e.g. not all Ketones are suffixed -ONE and not all Phenols are suffixed -OL, etc....

ARE ALL ESSENTIAL OILS SAFE TO USE?

Generally speaking essential oils are beneficial. However, it is not a truism to say because it is natural it is safe. Essential oils should always be used with care and caution! Some essential oils are highly toxic and should never be used in Aromatherapy. All Professional Aromatherapists should know this list of oils. Anyone considering using essential oils should check first with a qualified therapist.

It is a good idea to take a break from the daily use of the same oils at six weekly intervals.

If essential oils are being applied to the skin a period of at least twenty-four hours should be allowed to elapse between each full body massage. I believe two full Aromatherapy body massages per week to be sufficient.

As previously mentioned, certain oils should never be used for any conditions. In the interest of safety the therapist must also familiarise themself with the side effects of particular oils and when and where they must not be used.

Great care should be taken with pregnant women, children and the elderly; also those suffering with serious illnesses, contagious conditions, allergies, asthma, hayfever, rhinitis, sensitive skins and epilepsy as a number of oils are not recommended in these circumstances. Constant referral to text books and knowledge updated through professional therapists/organisations is a must for all who use essential oils.

SAFETY AND PRECAUTIONS

FIRE

Essential oils are flammable and should be kept away from naked flames. Materials (for example: couch roll or tissues used to mop up spillage of essential oils), should be put into an external waste bin. This material should not be put into the usual waste bins/area inside the work place. There is always the danger of a match, cigarette or hot candle being thrown into the bin or it being left near a source of heat.

ESSENTIAL OILS INTERNALLY INGESTED

No essential oil should be taken by mouth (ingested) unless prescribed by a medically qualified doctor. If essential oil is ingested by accident urgent medical advice should be sought.

POISONING

Prompt action is needed if an attempted overdose or an unknown amount of essential oil is ingested. Telephone the GP (doctor) or take the person to hospital without delay and bring the bottle along with you. If the person is unconscious telephone for an ambulance immediately and be sure you give the oil bottle to the ambulance crew. Do not attempt to induce vomiting unless advised to do so by a professional acting on medical guidance. The promptness of your action could save a life.

PATCH TESTING

How to do it : add 2 drops of essential oil to ½ teaspoon of carrier oil. Massage into inside of the upper arm and leave for six hours. If no reaction occurs then it is unlikely there will be a reaction to the oil. It is best to patch test new oils but there are no guarantees. If there is a reaction massage the area with lots of carrier oil especially if skin is sensitive or there is a tendency to allergies.

SPLASHES OF ESSENTIAL OIL INTO THE EYE

The eye should be washed immediately and bathed with lots of carrier/vegetable oil, milk or water; use an eyebath if possible and change the rinsing solution repeatedly. If the eye feels sore or continues to be painful get medical help.

SPLASHES OF ESSENTIAL OIL INTO THE MOUTH

Rinse the mouth out several times with carrier/vegetable oil, milk or water. If the inside of the mouth feels sore or painful seek medical advice. However, in most cases the latter step will not be necessary.

SPLASHES OF ESSENTIAL OIL ON THE SKIN

Wash the area thoroughly with carrier oil or milk. Normally this course of action should prevent any adverse reaction but obviously it will depend on the oil being used and the amount splashed on the skin.

VENTILATION

The therapist should try to ensure good ventilation between clients/treatments by opening the windows and doors for at least ten minutes. The therapist should try to spend this ten minutes in a different room where no oils are being used. Essential oils should not be burned continuously, particularly if there are young children or pets in the room.

SAFETY AND STORAGE

Always keep essential oils out of the reach of children. Use a locked cabinet or locked refrigerator. Do not leave oils in a normal household refrigerator where there is a danger of them being used by mistake (also the refrigerator will become impregnated with a strong essential oil smell). All essential oil for home use should have small neck stoppers/droppers as a precaution against children drinking the oil.

THERAPIST'S SAFETY

Results of over exposure of essential oils :-

Headaches, Limb Aches, Fatigue, Nausea, Itching, Red cheeks/hands.
Drinking a glass of water after each treatment helps to prevent a build up
of oils in the body and keep the therapist hydrated.

HAIR/GLASSES

If moving glasses up on your nose or pushing hair back off your face
while working use an arm instead of hands because your hands will
be covered in essential oil.

HANDS

Wash hands thoroughly before and after essential oil use.
Massage own hands, palms and backs, regularly with carrier oil,
especially at the end of the day.

LABELLING

All essential oil blended for home use should be clearly labelled, see
label example on page 73 and carry/display the following information:
External use only, Keep out of the reach of children, May irritate
skin if used undiluted, For use by named person only, Seek medical
advice if ingested, Name of essential oil(s) (Latin name), Use by
date, Name of therapist, Therapist contact details.

METHODS OF USING ESSENTIAL OILS IN AROMATHERAPY

MASSAGE

Massage is probably the most important and useful way to use essential oils in Aromatherapy. All the benefits of massage are difficult to measure. The oils work on the emotional as well as the physical plane. The interrelation between mind and body in massage is one of the main keys to its importance. Body massage relaxes not only muscles and improves lymph and blood flow it also helps to relieve tension and balance the body's energy flow. It promotes a feeling of well being and is believed by some to aid the absorption of oils into the skin. Aromatherapy massage should be considered to be a truly holistic therapy treating mind and body.

Each therapist has their own routine for massage. The variety of techniques is enormous but it really does not matter which method is used providing the therapist has had a thorough training. Most importantly the massage should physically encompass the whole body as the therapist takes into consideration the whole person, body and mind. Massage provides the therapist with the most effective way of introducing the oils into the body.

Massage improves lymph and blood flow thus bringing oxygen and nutrients to the tissues and removing waste products of cell metabolism.

In massage never use essential oils undiluted for the following reasons:

1. No slip
2. Highly concentrated
3. Could overdose (due to amount that would be needed)
4. Could cause damage (burn, rash or allergy)

COMPRESS

This is a very simple way of using essential oils especially when massage is contraindicated or if treating a specific condition such as a sprain, bruising, menstrual camp or rheumatism.

Prepare a container half full of either hot or cold water - a two litre container would have 10ml of blended oil added (6 drops of essential oil in 10ml of carrier). Soak a clean cloth in the preparation and then wring out the excess water. The cloth is then put on the area to be treated. Maximum benefit is gained by repeatedly soaking and wringing out the cloth and putting it on the affected area. Hot compresses are often used in chronic conditions, menstrual cramp and headaches caused through tension, especially if the back of the neck seems to be affected. Cold compresses seem to be more effective for reducing swelling and relieving pain; they can also be effective for some headaches. Compresses can be used on almost any area as it is easy to mold the material to the contours of the body including the face.

BATH

The majority of essential oils are not dispersed by water; the droplets stay on the top of the water. The benefits are gained by breathing in the odoriferous molecules. By blending the oils in a carrier and then adding them to the bath there is less danger of a reaction to the oil if used correctly. When undiluted oils are used in the bath no more than six drops should be used in the average bath (I do not recommend undiluted oils). No essential oil should ever be used in the bath without first checking suitability as some oil can cause skin irritation. If there is any doubt about skin sensitivity or allergies then test the oil in lower quantities first and gradually increase the drops to the recommended amount. In order to gain maximum benefit it is best to stay in the bath at least fifteen minutes; twenty minutes being an ideal length of time to soak. Cool baths are invigorating while warm baths have a calming effect. **Very hot baths** should be avoided, especially in cases of cardio-vascular conditions, during pregnancy and by those who are not physically very active. Hot baths are also very drying on the skin. Take extra care not to slip in an oily bath

Note ! Some modern baths may be stained by essential oil.

INHALATION OR STEAMING

Inhalation is an old remedy for colds and flu. It is another simple way to use the oils for a specific purpose ranging from chest to skin problems. Place one or two drops of pure essential oil in a bowl of boiling water. Before attempting this treatment ensure the bowl is secure on the table and one way to do this is to sit the bowl well back and resting on a wet/damp cloth (a damp cloth will prevent slip). When using a blended oil add 5 ml to the water).

Lean over the bowl with a large towel enclosing both your head and the bowl and inhale. The face should be about **twenty five centimetres (10 inches)** from the water and make sure to come out from under the towel every few minutes. **Begin** with about **half a minute** under the towel gradually building up to a few minutes. Breathing through the mouth helps sore throats, while breathing through the nose helps to unblock nasal passages. Once again, as with the bath oil, the properties of the oil should be checked. This treatment is sometimes offered by the professional therapist instead of, or prior to, another treatment; for example a facial massage, especially to clients suffering with sinusitis.

NOTE !

If you have sensitive skin especially with high pink/red colour or obvious thread veins, the first thing to do before preparing the inhalation is to cover the face with a thick layer of moisturiser or ointment base. Ideally this would be non-perfumed. It is also important to remember to **close your eyes** immediately you go under the towel.

VAPORISATION

The benefits and methods of evaporating essential oils seem endless. From placing a damp cloth, previously soaked in oil/water on the radiator to burning the oils in special burners or on ingeniously designed rings which fit onto lamp bulbs and containers that fit onto radiators. Oils used in this way can vary from Tea-Tree or Eucalyptus for 'flu bouts' to relaxing oils like Marjoram or Ylang-Ylang, Lavender and Chamomile through to 'wake me up' oils such as Rosemary and Peppermint. If using oils in the home then do consider the feelings of all the household. Do they all share the same needs?

ABSORPTION OF OILS

The molecular structure of the oil is very small, therefore some schools of thought believe that due to this fact the oil can be absorbed through the different layers of the skin and into the bloodstream. When essential oil molecules evaporate into the air they can be taken down into the lungs along with the air we breathe. Some will be exhaled in the next breath but some will pass, as oxygen does, into the bloodstream and travel around the body. As far as we know essential oils do not remain in the body but are passed out in exhalation, perspiration, urine and faeces.

Some books and therapists recommend essential oil to be taken by mouth. However, I believe that no essential oil should be taken orally unless prescribed by a medically qualified and recognised doctor. The oil must cope with the complex workings of the digestive system and the sensitive mucous membranes it encounters on its journey. There is the added danger of the essential oil having been adulterated and some oil may have a detrimental effect on the liver.

OILS - CARRIER OR BASE ?

Carrier oils are also known as Base or Fixed oils. Essential oils are mixed (blended) in a carrier oil before application to the skin. Fixed oils are non volatile, i.e. they evaporate extremely slowly.

The choice of carrier or base oil is governed by four main factors:

> 1. Smell
> 2. Texture
> 3. Price
> 4. Therapeutic value

In other words there should be little or no perfume. It should not be very sticky, should give good slip and preferably not be very expensive. Grapeseed and Sweet Almond oil are the most popular. The heavier, richer oils relatively speaking, are Avocado, Jojoba and Wheatgerm. Usually these three being used to enhance the quality of carrier oils, and are more usually used in percentages of between five and ten percent added to the main carrier.

NOTE !
Alcohol is sometimes used as a carrier, (e.g. Verruca treatment or perfume base).   I have chosen to suggest Vodka as a carrier for some of my recipes as it is more readily available for home use.

For those people who do not like to use alcohol then Jojoba oil is a useful alternative.

CARRIER OILS

ALMOND OIL (SWEET)
Skin   Dry, itching, inflamed,
                        sensitive.
                        It is obtained from the
                        kernel

Contains   Minerals, vitamins,
                        proteins and glucosides

Colour   Pale yellow

APRICOT KERNEL
Skin   Dry, dehydrated, inflamed
                        or mature. It is obtained
                        from the kernel

Contains   Minerals and vitamins

Colour   Pale yellow

CORN OIL
Skin   All skin types

Contains   Proteins, vitamins and
                        minerals

Colour   Pale yellow

GRAPESEED OIL

Skin

All skin types. Very light, almost odourless, therefore does not interfere with the aroma of the essential oil. It is also one of the least expensive carrier/ base oils

Contains

Vitamins, proteins and minerals

Colour

Pale green to colourless

HAZELNUT OIL

Skin

All skin types. This oil has a slightly astringent action. It is obtained from the kernel

Contains

Minerals, vitamins and proteins

Colour

Yellow

JOJOBA OIL

Skin

All skin types. Penetrates easily. It is especially good for acne, eczema, inflamed skins and psoriasis. This oil can feel a little sticky owing to its waxy substance, (mimics collagen) and is particularly useful for hairy skin

Many therapists will use the oil as a carrier for facial treatment; its penetrating powers makes it a useful oil when treating clients with a lot of subcutaneous tissue (fat)

Contains	Minerals and proteins
Colour	Yellow

OLIVE OIL

Uses	Mainly when rheumatic conditions are present and as a nourishing treatment for the hair. Disadvantage - it has a strong smell which is difficult to disguise
Contains	Minerals, vitamins and proteins
Colour	Green

SESAME OIL

Skin	Eczema, psoriasis. Other uses - arthritis, rheumatism, general aches and pains. Advantage - this oil washes out of clothing fairly easily, so indirectly could be considered the cheapest

Contains	Amino-acids, lecithin, minerals and vitamins
Colour	Dark yellow

SOYABEAN OIL / SAFFLOWER OIL

Skin	All skin types
Contains	Minerals, vitamins and proteins
Colour	All three oils are pale yellow

SUNFLOWER OIL

Skin	All skin types
Contains	Minerals and vitamins (no proteins)
Colour	Pale yellow

NOTE!
Ensure to check for nut allergies before using any nut oil.

OILS USED TO ENHANCE THE ACTION OF OTHER CARRIER OILS
USUALLY USED AS A 5% OR 10% DILUTION

AVOCADO

Skin

Dry, dehydrated or eczema. Very good penetrating powers; can be blended with other oils when treating areas of fatty tissue. Avocado is considered amongst the best nourishing oils. It is seldom used on its own which may be due in part to the high price of this oil.

Contains

Fatty acids, lecithin, proteins and vitamins

Colour

Dark green

CARROT OIL

Skin

Dry, ageing, itching, eczema, psoriasis. It also helps to reduce scarring. Carrot oil is often added to creams for facial treatments. Do not use undiluted on skin as it may turn the skin orange.

Contains

Beta-carotene, minerals and vitamins

Colour

Orange

EVENING PRIMROSE OIL

In its natural state the evening primrose is a wild flower. It is the newest of the wild plants to be grown as a crop. Strictly speaking it is not a primrose at all but belongs to the willow herb family. Evening Primrose is a fixed oil not a volatile oil.

Skin

All skin types but particularly sensitive, psoriasis, eczema and itching. Other uses P.M.T., Menopause, Heart disease, M.S. and Rheumatoid arthritis

Contains

Gamma linoleic acid, minerals and vitamins

Colour

Pale yellow

WHEATGERM OIL

Skin

All types especially dry and prematurely ageing as well as for eczema and psoriasis. It is also considered as an anti-scarring agent due to the vitamin E content. As it is a very sticky oil it offers little lubrication. Therefore for use as a carrier it is best in proportions of 25% wheatgerm to 75% of other base carrier oil

Contains

Minerals, proteins and vitamins

Colour

Yellow/Orange

BLENDING GUIDE

Blending code for essential oil therapy.

5ml equals 100 drops, approximately 1 teaspoon. Therefore when blending essential oils the following guide should be applied:

¼% =   1 drop essential oil in 20ml (or 400 drops) carrier

½% =   1 drop essential oil in 10ml (or 200 drops) carrier

1% =   1 drop essential oil in 5ml (or 100 drops) carrier

2% =   2 drops essential oil in 5ml (or 100 drops) carrier

2½%=   5 drops essential oil in 10ml (or 200 drops) carrier

3% =   3 drops essential oil in 5ml (or 100 drops) carrier

The drops can only be an approximate measure as drop size will differ according to the dispenser and the viscosity of the oil, (for accuracy it is advisable to purchase a suitably marked measurer).

To prepare an Aromatherapy blend add the required number of drops to a clean, dry, empty bottle and then add the carrier (oil, alcohol, etc). Put the cap on tightly. Wipe the bottle and label it. Slowly turn the bottle upside down and back five times. Store in a cool place ready for use.

A therapist could prepare basic blends of individual oil and carrier on a weekly or even fortnightly basis. This is easily done if the average massage blending at 2% or 2½% is adhered to.

They can prepare the commonly used oils in 50ml bottles.
The less commonly used oils in 25ml bottles and the stronger or least used oils in 10ml bottles.

If oils are being prepared in this way the therapist should take some measures to protect themself from a buildup of oils:

1. Wear protective clothing (overall)
2. Wear polythene gloves
3. Wear a face mask
4. Wear protective eye wear - glasses or swimming goggles
5. Wear a hat or head band to avoid having to push hair off the face (touching face with a gloved hand)
6. If you wear glasses and feel the need to reposition them on your nose, push them up using the forearm, not the hand
7. Wash their hands thoroughly
8. Drink lots of water once the task is finished

When making products (face creams/toners/moisturisers) for daily use it is wise to keep the amount of essential oil to minimum percentages; as a general guide this could be in the region of 0.005 percent. It is unwise to be subjected daily to oils in skin products, baths/showers, vaporisers and massage. According to the well known saying 'You can have too much of a good thing'.

TOP, MIDDLE AND BASE NOTES
WHAT DO THEY MEAN?

To the more modern Aromatherapist the notes are merely a guide. The idea of classification in this manner is taken from the world of the perfumer and in that context is taken to mean a distinctive odour effect which can be identified and named. The idea was devised by a nineteenth century Italian, Septimus Piesse. He compared odours with sounds. Scents, he said, appear to influence the olfactory nerves in certain definite degrees. There is, as it were, an octave of odours like an octave in music. Certain odours coincide like the keys of an instrument. To each note Piesse assigned a note of the musical scale and to each note he assigned the odour of a natural source: middle C for example, corresponded to Camphor, and so on. He believed that in order to create a harmonious perfume the odours appearing in his listings should be blended together to correspond with a cord formed from the respective musical notes (this method of blending perfumes no longer applies).

In perfume the top note is the first to be observed it is the most volatile, lasting only between 10-30 minutes gradually giving way to the middle (or heart) note, which is the main fragrance of the perfume. This mixture is maintained with the support of a mixture from low volatile base notes.

The base notes slow down the volatility rate of the top and middle notes (they "fix" other essences). Therefore they are always used in perfume for their staying power. Two of the most commonly used fixatives (base notes) are Sandalwood and Patchouli.

When an essential oil evaporates we have a constantly changing composition which in turn gives a constantly changing odour. However the change is hardly noticeable as we continually smell the odour.

The theory of blending essential oils by note does have its faults as not all experts are in agreement as to which oils are top, middle and base. In view of these differences in Perfumery and Aromatherapy many Aromatherapists ignore the old perfumers' method of blending oils.

When blending essential oils by note it is usual to blend a top note plus a middle or base note. The top note is the most volatile and fast acting with an uplifting aroma which is relatively short lived. The middle note is moderately volatile, uplifting and relaxing. The base note is the least volatile of the oils, relaxing with a long lasting aroma.

EVAPORATION

Evaporation simply means the change from liquid or solid to vapour.

The evaporation of a solid to vapour without first melting is called sublimation: in other words the solid slowly disappears over a period of time.

A typical example of evaporation, as we have all observed, is the drying up of a puddle of water. It is worth noting that the evaporation of alcohol and of water takes place much faster than the evaporation of an essential oil.

VOLATILITY

This could be simply explained as:
1. The speed (rate) of evaporation
2. The time taken for the odour of an oil to become undetectable under controlled conditions
3. Essential oils readily disappear in the open air. They are volatile

SHELF LIFE OF ESSENTIAL OILS BLENDED AND UNBLENDED

Essential oils evaporate very readily. They are damaged by exposure to air, light, heat, cold and moisture, in fact any temperature changes and extremes. They should be stored in tightly closed dark glass bottles.

Essential oils, in theory, should last for years but the more often they are exposed to air by opening the greater the chance of oxidation, which will reduce the therapeutic value of the oil and possibly cause skin reaction. As a general guide, citrus oils have the shortest shelf life, about nine months to one year whilst other oils will usually last about two years, though it is said that Frankincense and Sandalwood improve with age. As essential oils deteriorate there is a detectable change in aroma; they become more cloudy in appearance and may show colour change. Essential oils unopened should be used within a two year period if stored in ideal conditions and within a one year period from being opened. As previously mentioned there is a risk of getting skin reaction from oils that have been subjected to degradation, i.e. chemical changes occurring due to light, heat and atmospheric oxygen (photocatalytic reaction refers to deterioration due to light). Do not use essential oils if sold/kept in clear bottles. For storage pour small amounts from large bottles into small bottles.

BLENDED OILS

Once the essential oils are blended (and opened for use), their shelf life is reduced to just three or four months, (less if conditions are not ideal). The lifespan can be prolonged for a little longer with the addition of vitamin E oil which has antioxidant properties. Some therapists add a small percentage (5%) of wheatgerm oil to blends as it is believed to have antioxidant properties but I find when used for this purpose it does little more than stain the towel and uniforms.

PURCHASE AND STORAGE

If buying a pre-blended oil from a retail outlet it would be a wise precaution to ask the following questions:

1. Date the oil was blended?

2. If oils are purchased pre-blended or blended on site?

3. Under what conditions the oils are stored?

4. What percentage of essential oil is contained in the carrier?

Remember during the purchase and sell on process essential oils often pass through several hands before ending up on the shop shelf. If in doubt buy well known brand names available direct from the supplier or chosen outlets.

Purchase date and storage details may also be queried on pure, non-blended essential oils.

NOTE !
A number of the oils being sold for use in vaporisers are synthetic. They are not true essential oils or absolutes.

All aromatherapy oils should be stored in a cool place. Those of citrus and herb origin are best kept in a refrigerator, (kept solely for the purpose of oil storage) at about 5°C. The wood oils keep as much as possible at a constant room temperature of 15°C. The resinoids and gums will keep in a cool place (garage or basement).

Try to purchase oils in small quantities. If you are unlikely to use more than 10ml of a particular oil every six months it is pointless to purchase 20ml. If, however, through circumstance it is necessary for you to purchase for example 20ml at a time then perhaps it would be possible for you to share the cost and the quantity with a colleague. Divide the supply into four 5ml bottles and label each bottle with:

1.   The name of the oil - Botanical
2.   The date of purchase
3.   The supplier

Then take two bottles each, one for regular use and the other for storage. Alternatively keep three bottles in your cool dark storage area and bottle number four for your regular use.

Each time the bottle is opened some of the top note vapour will escape and at the same time air will get into the bottle bringing with it a new oxygen supply. By choosing and using the smallest sized bottle of essential oil the amount of air in contact with the oil (in the bottle) is kept to a minimum, therefore helping to ensure the quality of the oil used. Make sure all essential oil bottles have a small tight fitting dropper fitted in the neck as this will reduce the possibility of air getting to the oil as well as reducing the risk of accidental spillage or consumption

When the essential oil bottle is empty or partly empty do not be tempted to refill this bottle with a fresh supply of oil as the fresh oil will become contaminated by the deteriorating dregs of the previous oil (some suppliers ask that their bottles be returned when empty).

I wash all my empty bottles in a solution of vinegar, Tea-Tree oil and salt, before placing them in the dishwasher. If you do not have a dishwasher then wash with suggested solution followed by a short (10 minute) soak in a solution of Epsom Salts (5 grams to 1 litre).

NOTE !
Epsom Salts can help the removal of any oil smell and/or stain from towels and clothing.

PURCHASE, SALES AND LABELLING

Example of purchase book entry :-

Date	Supplier	Product	Quantity	Cost	Comment
1/12/99	ML Gad	Jasmine	5 ml	£	Kept
5/12/99	Hadwell	Tangerine	5 ml	£	Returned

Example of sales book entry :-

Date	Name/Address	Tel. No.	Condition/Symptom	Quantity Sold

Base Oil %	Essential Oil %	Instructions for Use	Total Charge

Example of label information :-

Date Blended	Name of Client	Carrier Oil	Essential Oil	Storage Instructions	Expiry Date

Safety Instructions	Instructions For Use	Therapist Details	Use by

SEEK MEDICAL ADVICE IF INGESTED / MAY IRRITATE SKIN IF UNDILUTED

KEEP OUT OF THE REACH OF CHILDREN

73

CARRIAGE NOTES

Today	**Yesteryear**
Glass bottles	Alabaster pots
Stainless steel	Onyx pots
Aluminium	Wooden pots

Stainless steel drums with lacquered interiors are used in transportation and for large quantity storage of essential oils.

Aluminium drums internally lacquered are used for storage and transportation of small amounts.

Plastic can be used for very short periods only as the essential oil will attack and break down the plastic; hence there will be a detrimental effect on the essential oil. Special double plastic bottles are now being used for pre blended oils, available through good retailers.   (I personally prefer glass).

It is important to note that the containers used for the storage of essential oils should be made of a material that will not allow air or light to the oil and will not cause any chemical interaction with the oil.

NOTE !
The only time I will blend oils in small quantities into strong plastic bottles for home use is for my blind or frail clients when there may be a danger of dropping the glass bottle with dangerous consequences or other times when I need to advise spray use as in athlete's foot.

THE ESSENTIAL OIL PROFILES

THE CHEMICAL COMPONENTS OF THE ESSENTIAL OIL

A typical essential oil contains several hundred individual chemicals with the great majority at levels of less then one percent. I have endeavoured to add some of the main known chemical constituents of each oil, however it should be noted that the main chemical components do not necessarily contribute to the recognised odour of the oil.

TRACE COMPONENTS

Sometimes the trace elements are so low in concentration as not to be detected by gas chromatography but can still be smelled in essential oil. In a number of citrus oils Thymol and Eugenol are present only as traces and yet contribute distinctly to their odour. These trace components probably contribute significantly to the therapeutic effects of the essential oil, just as they do to the odour.

THE PROPERTIES OF ESSENTIAL OIL

Each essential oil is credited with numerous properties and this can be a minefield for students when trying to decide which oil to use.

In the individual oil profile laid out in the following pages I have attempted to give some of the properties which may be helpful for memory and choice.

I have expanded on the properties listing on page 246. As all essential oils have to a greater or lesser extent some antiseptic properties I have omitted this from the individual profiles.

NOTE !

I have offered suggestions on some of the more common usage for each oil.

ODOUR

In each individual profile I have added a general impression of odour relative to that pure essential oil but smell is a very individualistic interpretation without a true language of its own. When the oil is mixed with a carrier the odour will change; when different oils are blended together the odour changes yet again. The final mixture must have a smell that is pleasing to the recipient, otherwise I do not believe it will be as effective in use as intended.

ADULTERATION

I have included some information on the subject of adulteration relative to each individual essential oil. I would hope oils purchased from reputable suppliers would be as expected for standard of quality.

However, the only way to guarantee the essential oil quality would be to collect it from the still, having observed the entire process, and even then it could not be guaranteed that there were no biocides in the oil.

SYNERGIES

Madam Maury called it "Individual Prescription", oils chosen in a balance to treat physical and emotional requirements, the condition, temperament and circumstance having been considered. Odour and oils will blend harmoniously playing a part in the success of the outcome. In other words to have synergy is to have total balance.

CAUTION

To each oil profile I have added a heading **CAUTION** where I advise caution relative to an individual condition and oil. I have not been specific in separating methods of use or percentages of oil likely to be more at fault in use. It is not within the remit of this book to give an in-depth breakdown on each oil and it is recommended that where such information is required more specialised technical reading be undertaken.

Instead I have brought the possible negative aspects of the oil to the attention of the reader. In general, toxicity is dose dependent; the more of a substance used the greater the potential for harm. Toxic reactions depend not only on the amount used but also on the method of use and the physiological status of the client/patient.

ILLUSTRATIONS

The plants, trees, flowers, fruits and roots relative to the individual oils are the artist's representation of the plant material.

BASIL

Note	Top
Botanical Name	Ocimum Basilicum (Sweet Basil)
Family	Labiatae
Cultivation	France, (Mediterranean) Asia
Part of Plant	Flowering tops and leaves
Extracted by	Steam Distillation
Yield 1 Gram Oil	Equals 2000 grams of base material
Constituents	**Alcohol** - Linalool **Keytones** - Borneone **Oxide** - Cineole **Phenols** - Methylchavicol Eugenol **Pinene** - Sylvestrene **Terpenes** - Ocimene
Principal Constituents	Linalool, Methylchavicol Cineole. Small amounts of many other constituents are also found in the oil French Basil (Sweet Basil) low in Methylchaviol and high in Linalool
Adulteration	Sweet Basil, with synthetic Linalool and other types of Basil

Colour	Pale yellow
Aroma	Spicy
Blends well with	Geranium, Bergamot, Lavender, Clary-Sage, Sandalwood
Properties	Emmenagogue, Insecticide, Stimulant

MOST COMMON USES

Respiratory	Chest infections, Asthma, Bronchitis, Catarrh
Digestive	Indigestion, Flatulance
Muscular	Tired, overworked muscles
Other	Insect repellant, wasp sting, mosquito bite

METHODS OF USE	Inhaler, Vaporiser, Bath, Massage
CAUTION	Methychavicol is a suspected skin sensitiser.

IMPORTANT NOTE !
These oils should not exceed 2% dilution for any treatment and always ensure that the oil being used is low in Methylchavicol

BASIL

An annual herb which grows to approximately 20cm in height.
The erect stems have numerous branches bearing opposite, stalked, broadly ovate and pointed leaves. These leaves are pale green in colour and bear purple ornaments. Oil glands are dotted along the leaf. The herb flowers in the summer producing white flowers sometimes with a purple tinge.

NOTE !
High doses are believed by some to be potentially carcinogenic.
I do not use Basil oil in my clinic.

BASIL

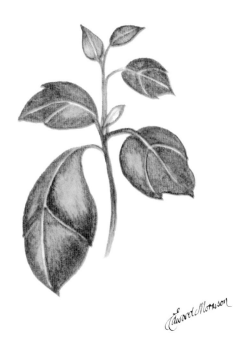

Ocimum Basilicum

BENZOIN

Note	Base
Botanical Name	Styrax Benzoin
Family	Styracaceae
Cultivation	Java, Sumatra, Thailand
Part of Plant	Gum from tree
Extracted by	Steam distillation
Yield 1 Gram Oil	Equals 15 grams base material
Constituents	**Acids** - Benzoic, Cinnamic **Aldehydes** - Benzoic aldehyde (Benzaldehyde), Vanillin **Esters** - Benzyl benzoate
Principal Constituents	Benzyl benzoate, Benzoic acid, Cinnamic acids
Adulteration	Unlikely
Colour	Yellow/reddish brown
Aroma	Sweet/ vanilla

Blends well with	Sandalwood, Rose, Jasmine
Properties	Carminative, Deodorant, Sedative

MOST COMMON USES

Respiratory	Bronchitis, Coughs, Asthma
Musculoskeletal	Arthritis, Rheumatism
Other	Gout, Colic, Sedative

METHODS OF USE	Compress, Local massage
CONTRA INDICATIONS	Children
CAUTION	Can be a skin sensitiser

NOTE !
May cause cross sensitivity to other oils, especially gums, resins and balsams.

BENZOIN

The Benzoin tree's main habitat is Java and Sumatra. This large tree grows to about 60ft. (20m) in height. The leaves are pale green on top and whitish underneath. The tree does not produce Benzoin in the normal course of events. It is a pathological product obtained only after the infliction of a wound sufficiently severe to injure the bark and trunk. The tree then exudes or accumulates beneath the bark the liquid Benzoin. When the Benzoin hardens the tears (droplets) are collected.

The first incisions are made when the tree is seven years old. The tree continues to produce in this way for a further ten or so years with the finest quality being produced in the first three years. The final year's supply is obtained when the tree is felled and its contents scraped out.

Benzoin is firstly extracted with Benzene before being subject to steam distillation.

BENZOIN

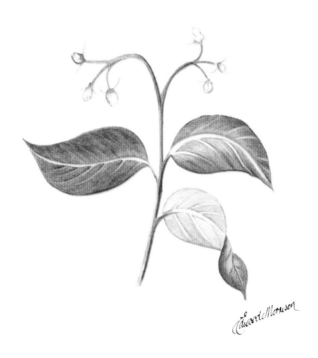

Styrax Benzoin

BERGAMOT

Note	Top
Botanical Name	Citrus Bergamia
Family	Rutaceae
Cultivation	Italy, Morocco (West Africa)
Part of Plant	Rind of fruit
Extracted by	Expression
Yield 1 Gram Oil	Equals 200 grams base material
Constituents	**Alcohols** - Linalool, Nerol & Terpineol **Ester** - Linalyl acetate **Lactone** - Bergaptene **Terpenes** - Dipentene, Limonene
Principal Constituents	Linalyl acetate, Limonene Over 300 components in expressed oil including Furacoumarines, mainly Bergaptene.
Adulteration	Bitter Orange oil, Lime oil, synthetic Linalool, Linalyl acetate, Limonene and others.

Colour	Green
Aroma	Citrus
Blends well with	Cypress, Jasmine, Lavender, Neroli, Ylang-Ylang, Chamomile, Marjoram
Properties	Analgesic, Antidepressant, Anti-Inflammatory, Antiseptic, Bactericide

MOST COMMON USES

Emotional	Tension/Anxiety, Depression, Anorexia Nervosa
Urinary	Urinary tract infections, Urethritis, Cystitis, Vaginal Pruritus
Skin	Acne, Infected, Oily
Other	Insect Repellent, Room freshener, Inhibits certain viruses, Herpes Simplex, Herpes Zoster (shingles), Chickenpox

METHODS OF USE   Bath, Compress, Massage, Vaporiser

CAUTION

Allow 12 hours before and after exposure to UV (sun/sun bed).
Results of exposure to UV and Bergaptene are redness, burning, irregular hyperpigmented patches.

The chemical **Bergaptene** (plus 8 other furanocoumarins) are responsible for increasing photosensitivity of the skin. Bergaptene free Bergamot (fractioned oil) is available and does not effect the skin (do check oil and client suitability). These oils are referred to as F.C.F oils.

BERGAMOT

The Bergamot tree grows to 15ft (4.5m). The leaves are long and green and the flowers white. The tree bears yellow, small, almost pear-shaped fruit. Harvest time is from December to February.

The main countries producing the oil are Italy and Sicily and to a lesser extent Africa. The oil has a long history and has been mentioned in many old herbals and manuscripts.

One of my favourite uses for this beautiful green oil is in the room vaporiser. I also tend to use it for most of the conditions mentioned overleaf. I tend not to use the oil on the skin in the summer months as skin reactions can occur when the skin is exposed to ultra violet light either from the sun or the use of a sunbed. In the winter months I do use the oil after warning my clients about U.V. exposure (sun or sunbeds).

I do not use this oil if the skin shows signs of Melanoma, Pre-Melanoma, large dark moles or any skin Cancers.

BERGAMOT

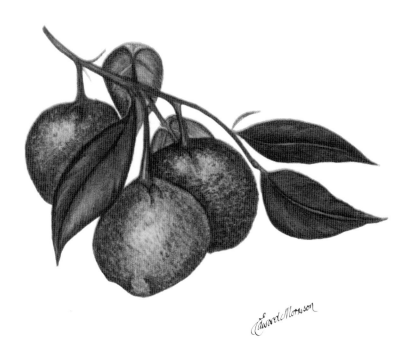

Citrus Bergamia

BLACKPEPPER

Note	Middle
Botanical Name	Piper Nigrum
Family	Piperaceae
Cultivation	Singapore, Sumatra, Penang, (East Asia)
Part of Plant	Unripe berries
Extracted by	Steam distillation
Yield 1 Gram Oil	Equals 50 grams base material
Constituents	**Phenols -** Safrole **Sesquiterpene -** Caryophyllene, Bisabolene, Farnesene **Terpenes -** Camphene, Limonene, Myrcene, Phellandrene, Pinene, Sabinene, Selinene, Thugene
Principal Constituents	Thugene, Pinene, Camphene
Adulteration	Occasionally with Pennyroyal or other peppermints.
Colour	Colourless/pale green/pale yellow
Aroma	Freshly ground peppercorns/warm

Blends well with	Frankincense, Rosemary, Sandalwood, Marjoram, Lavender, Ylang-Ylang
Properties	Analgesic, Rubefacient, Digestive, Stimulant

MOST COMMON USES

Digestive	Colic, Indigestion, Constipation
Musculoskeletal	Aches, Pains, Rheumatic, Arthritic, Athletes' aches and pains

METHODS OF USE	Compress, Local massage
CAUTION	Use at a maximum 1% in hypersensitive individuals, (due to rubefacient properties). Slightly phototoxic, avoid blending with known phototoxic oils.

BLACK PEPPER

The Pepper is a native of Asia. In the cultivated state the creeping vine grows to about 10-12ft (3-4m) in height but if left untouched the vine can reach 20ft (6m) in height. Only at three to four years old will the vine begin to produce peppers which it will then continue to produce at the rate of about 4lb a year for a further 15 years.

The leaves are dark green, the flowers small and white.

Pepper has been mentioned in many of the great scripts throughout history; Chinese in the twelfth century, Theophrastus and Pliny. Pepper was one of the spices that inspired the voyages of exploration.

I find that to use this oil sparingly gives me good results (I have only ever used it locally). My favourite uses for the oil are: Muscular stiffness/fatigue prior to or directly after running or dancing; also on local areas of rheumatic pain.

BLACK PEPPER

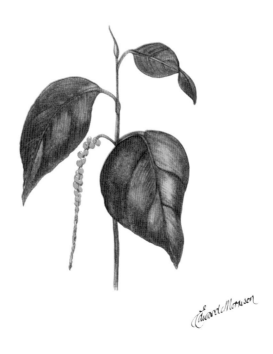

Piper Nigrum

CAJUPUT

Note	Top
Botanical Name	Melaleuca Leucodendron
Family	Myrtaceae
Cultivation	Malaysia (Far East)
Part of Plant	Leaves/Buds
Extracted by	Steam distillation
Yield 1 Gram Oil	Equals 65 grams base material
Constituents	**Alcohol** - Terpineol **Aldehyde** - Benzaldehyde **Oxide** - Cineole **Terpenes** - Pinene, Limonene, Dipentene
Principal Constituent	Cineole
Adulteration	Can be replaced by cheaper Eucalyptus oils, (not necessarily globulus) and/or traces of terpinol acetate, propionate esters.

Colour	Pale yellow/pale green
Aroma	Camphorous
Blends well with	Peppermint, Geranium, Lavender, Niaouli, Rose
Properties	Antineuralgic, Antirheumatic, Decongestant, Insecticide

MOST COMMON USES

Respiratory System	Colds/Flu, Respiratory Infections
Skin	Can be beneficial for some skin conditions such as Psoriasis and Acne
METHOD OF USE	Inhalation, Local massage
CAUTION	Oil is a mild rubefacient and as a result it is included in a number of liniments and ointments.

CAJUPUT

The Cajuput tree is found in Australia, Malaysia and East India. The tree is a tall evergreen that can reach a height of 4Oft (13.5m) with thick pointed leaves and white flowers. The Cajuput tree is sometimes referred to as the 'crooked white tree' which is probably due to the fact that both the trunk and irregular branches have a white scaly bark which is easy to remove.

The leaves, twigs and buds are fermented before distillation.

The oil was used by the Malay and Indonesian peoples for its therapeutic properties long before its appearance in Europe in the mid 1600's.

In my opinion there are two reasons why the use of Cajuput should be left to the professional:
1. Cajuput can be a skin irritant
2. Cajuput is sometimes adulterated with other oils. The professional therapist can always check quality with his/her supplier.

As Cajuput is a powerful stimulant it should be used in the evening only if it is blended with a sedative oil such as Chamomile.

The most common use I have for the oil is in a room burner or house spray when there is flu about. I have often used it this way to treat sinusitis.

CAJUPUT

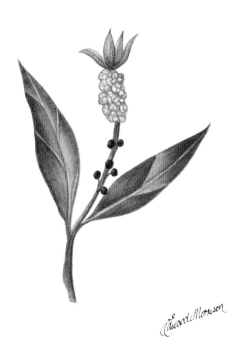

Melaleuca Leucodendron

CEDARWOOD

Note	Base
Botanical Name	Cedrus Atlantica
Family	Cupresaceae
Cultivation	North Africa (Morocco)
Part of Plant	Wood
Extracted by	Steam distillation
Yield 1 Gram Oil	Equals 30 grams of base material
Constituents	**Alcohol** - Cedrol, Cedrenol **Sequiterpenes** - Cadinene, Cedrene **Terepene** - Thujopsene
Principal Constituents	Cedrol, Cedrene, Thujopsene
Adulteration	With other cedarwood oils including Texas Cedarwood, which is of a different family.

Colour	Yellow
Aroma	Woody/cedar
Blends well with	Bergamot, Cypress, Jasmine, Neroli, Rosemary, Juniper, Lavender, Rose
Properties	Astringent, Expectorant, Fungicide, Insecticide

MOST COMMON USES

Respiratory	Infections, Catarrah, Coughs
Skin	Acne, Dandruff, Scalp disorders, Insect repellent
Other	Urinary infections, Cystitis, Vaginal infections

METHOD OF USE	Bath, Massage, Inhalation
CAUTION	Due to adulteration it may cause skin irritation especially on hypersensitive individuals.

CEDARWOOD

If Jasmine and Rose are considered to be the King and Queen of the oils and flowers surely the title of King of the trees and forests should be bestowed on this tall majestic evergreen that grows to about 100ft (30m) commanding space for its expansive branches.

The needles form in rosette bunches with barrel shaped upright cones and yellow flowers.

The Cedarwood can live for well over a thousand years. The wood is very aromatic and resists attack from insects; perhaps this is one reason why it was chosen by the Egyptians to build their ships, furniture and coffins, (the oil was used in mummification). The Temple of Solomon was built with Cedarwood. It is still used as a temple incense by the Tibetans. Today the Red Cedarwood (Juniperous Virginiana) tends to be used for making smaller items such as pencils.

I use this oil in burners and sprays as an insect repellent, for chronic conditions such as arthritis/rheumatism and as a fixative for my perfumes.

CEDARWOOD

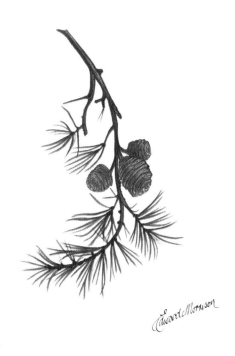

Cedrus Atlantica

CHAMOMILE

Note	Middle
Botanical Name	Roman - Anthemis Nobilis German - Matricaria Chamomilla
Family	Compositae
Cultivation	Roman - Belgium, England, Morocco German - Hungary, Russia
Part of Plant	Flowers
Extracted by	Steam distillation
Yield 1 Gram Oil	Equals 100 grams base material
Constituents	**Roman:** **Acids** - Tiglic, Methacrylic, Angelic **Aldehyde** - Cunnnic **Sesquiterpene** - Azuline **German:** **Sesquiterpene** - Azuline
Principal Constituents	Roman: Angelic, Tigilic acids German: Chamazulene, Farnesene
Adulteration	Nobilis - Mixed with or completely substituted for cheaper Moroccan oil.
Matricaria	Synthetic Chamazulene added particularly to aging/old oil to enhance the colour, (old oil will turn green/brown). Cheaper Moroccan oil substituted for Matricia after addition of colour enhancing synthetic Chamazulene.

Colour	**Roman** - Pale blue, greenish blue to yellow. **German** - Deep blue (due to azulene)
Aroma	Sharp / apple-like
Blends well with	Most oils, particularly Geranium, Lavender, Patchouli, Rose, Neroli, Ylang-Ylang, Jasmine, Marjoram
Properties	Anticonvulsive, Antidepressant, Antiemetic, Anti-inflammatory, Sedative.
CAUTION	Those who suffer with pollen allergy should exercise caution in the use of this oil.

NOTE !
Matricia (German Oil) has a much stronger anti-inflamatory reaction due to the high azulene content.

MOST COMMON USES

Digestive	Diarrhoea, Flatulence, Indigestion, Stomach ulcers
Gynaecological	Menstrual irregularity, Menopausal symptoms
Neurological	Neuralgia
Emotional	Anxiety, Depression, Insomnia
Skin	Acne, Thread veins, Mature, Dry, Burns
Other	Ear ache, Toothache

Like Lavender, Chamomile is one of the most versatile oils

METHODS OF USE   Bath, Compress, Massage, Inhalation, Vapourizer

NOTE !
Do not put drops directly into ear.

CHAMOMILE - ANTHEMIS NOBILIS

Cultivated mainly in Europe the plant grows up to 12 inches (30cm) high. It has a deep root and produces several stems, some erect and some branched.

The leaves are pinnately divided into short and mainly hairy leafets. The flowers are arranged in terminal stemmed white ray flower heads, resembling the daisy. Flowering time is mid Summer to early Autumn.

CHAMOMILE - MATRICARIA

A native of Europe and North West Africa this is an annual plant very similar to the Nobilis. The plant forms a clump with several erect smooth stems bearing finely divided hairless leaves and a solitary daisy-like flower head. The flower head has an outer ray of white florets surrounding an inner yellow disk. The flower head of the Matricaria is much smaller than that of the Nobilis.

GENERAL

The qualities and properties of both oils overlap. The Matricaria is much more blue and ink-like in colour.

Chamomile was considered sacred by the Egyptians and was used as a disinfectant in hospitals up to the Second World War. Some of the great herbalists of the past made claims for its uses which are still accepted today.

One of my favourite oils for complaints such as facial neuralgia, sinusitis, PMT and indigestion. It is also a good oil to use for childhood problems such as sleeplessness, earache, tummy ache and diarrhoea.

CHAMOMILE GERMAN

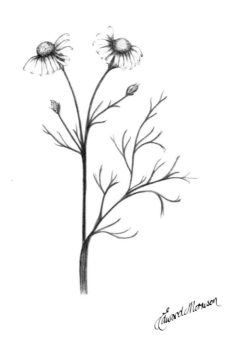

Matricaria Chamomilla

CHAMOMILE ROMAN

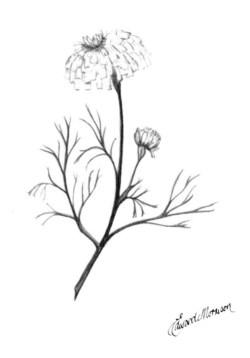

Anthemis Nobilis

CINNAMON LEAF

Note	Top
Botanical Name	Cinnamomum Zeylanicum
Family	Lauraceae
Cultivation	Sri Lanka, China, Madagascar
Part of Plant	Leaf (also a bark essence)
Extracted by	Steam distillation
Yield 1 Gram	Equals 50 grams of base material
Constituents	**Alcohol** - Linalool **Phenol** - Eugenol, Safrol
Principal Constituents	Eugonol
Adulteration	May be mixed with Clove Bud oil or Bay Leaf oil and or synthetic Eugonol.
Colour	Yellow
Aroma	Spicy/ Warm/ Strong

Blends well with	Florals, Woods, Lemongrass, Mandarin, Myrrh, Benzoin
Properties	Antidepressant, Aphrodisiac, Hypotensive Uterine Tonic, Sedative

MOST COMMON USES

Skin	Scabies, Lice, Boils
Circulation	Stimulates sluggish circulation
Digestive	Sluggish digestion, Flatulence, Colic, Digestive spasms, Diarrhoea
Respiratory	Colds, Coughs, Sore throats, Chills/aches due to fever, Sinusitis
Mental States	Depression, Nervous exhaustion, Fatigue
METHODS OF USE	Massage, Vaporiser, Inhaler
CAUTION	Kidney, Liver, Lupus, Cancer, Haemophilia disorders. Also for those taking anticoaglant drugs or regular Paracetamol users. Sensitive skin (can be an irritant) May irritate mucous membrane.

NOTE !
Cinnamon Leaf oil must not be confused with Cinnamon Bark oil which is a hazardous oil and should not be used in Aromatherapy.

CINNAMON LEAF

The trees grow in tropical climates up to a height of 15m. The leaves are shiny green with a leathery feel producing a spicy smell when brushed.

The berries are oval shaped and blue in colour while the flowers are small and white in colour.

The bark is scab like and when new shoots become visible they are speckled orange and green. The cinnamon is a very old and respected spice.

The Egyptians used the spice for bathing the feet and for ridding the body of excessive bile. The Chinese used it to normalise abdominal gas and to balance the temperature of the liver.

The Greeks used it for its great antiseptic properties and the Europeans have used Cinnamon as a love potion, as an aid to childbirth and since the 9th century as an ingredient in mulled wine.

I use it as an antiseptic and for digestive disorders.

CINNAMON LEAF

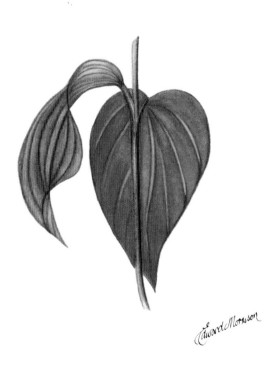

Cinnamomum Zeylanicum

CLARY SAGE

Note	Top/Middle
Botanical Name	Salvia Sclarea
Family	Labiatae
Cultivation	France, Russia, Morocco, Italy
Part of Plant	Flowering tops and foliage
Extracted by	Steam distillation
Yield 1 Gram Oil	Equals 800 grams base material
Constituents	**Alcohol** - Salviol, Linalool **Ester** - Linalyl acetate **Sesquiterpene -** Caryophyllene **Oxide**-Cineole
Principal Constituents	Lynalyl acetate, Linalool Over 250 component trace elements that contribute to the odour
Adulteration	Lavender, Bergamot mint (mentha citrata). Synthetic - Linalyl acetate and Linalool.
Colour	Colourless/ pale yellowish.
Aroma	Sweet/ Muscatel wine-like

Blends well with	Cedarwood, Citrus, Geranium, Frankincense, Jasmine, Juniper, Lavender, Sandalwood
Properties	Antidepressant, Antispasmodic, Hypotensive, Uterine Tonic, Sedative

MOST COMMON USES

Emotional	Mental fatigue, Stress
Respiratory	Asthma, Sore throats
Circulatory	High blood pressure
Gynaecological	Menstrual problems, Infertility
Skin	Mature

METHOD OF USE	Bath, Compress, Massage, Perfume, Vapouriser
CAUTION	May cause mucous membrane irritation / sensitisation in some hypersensitive individuals.

NOTE !

Reported to cause nightmares if used immediately prior to or after alcohol consumption. It is also reported to have oestrogenic qualities but this claim still lacks full scientific proof.

CLARY SAGE

A native to southern Europe though now cultivated worldwide.
Dry soil is important (damp soil rots the roots). The plant tends to hug the ground but can grow to 3ft (90cm). The leaves are large and grey-green in colour; they are heart shaped, wrinkled and pointed and are covered with velvety hairs. The flowers are blue or white and bloom in August.

Clary Sage has many similar properties to Sage. One of its greater benefits is that it contains a far lower proportion of Thujone and therefore does not present the risk of toxicity associated with Sage.

Both Sage and Clary Sage have a long history and were mentioned by Hypocrites, Dioscorides, Romans, Egyptians and the Herbals of the Middle Ages.

In Germany, Clary Sage was called Muscatel Sage and was used by some wine makers to enhance the flavour of cheap wines, (makes them taste like true Muscatel). The results were, it is said, an exaggerated state of drunkenness.

Warning - Clary Sage should not be used on or by anybody who has consumed or is about to consume alcohol as this can cause drowsiness and in some cases severe nightmares.

Clary Sage is a very relaxing oil for the physical and emotional state; it should therefore be used with caution on people who are expected to have great mental clarity or to drive home after a treatment.

Clary Sage is one of my favourite oils for the treatment of asthmatics and also for the treatment of abdominal cramp whether caused through digestive or menstrual problems.

CLARY SAGE

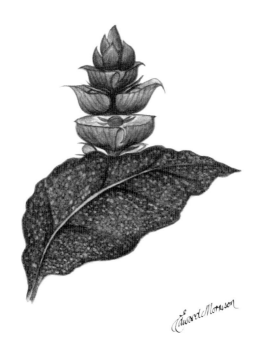

Salvia Sclarea

CYPRESS

Note	Middle/Base
Botanical Name	Cupressus Sempervirens
Family	Cupressaceae
Cultivation	France, Germany
Part of Plant	Leaves, Cones
Extracted by	Steam distillation
Yield 1 Gram Oil	Equals 150 grams base material
Constituents	**Alcohol** - Sabinol **Ester** - Terpenyl acetate **Terpenes** - Camphene, Cymene, Pinene, Sylvestrene
Principal Constituents	Pinene, Camphene
Adulteration	May be mixed with cheaper oil from other Cupressus species.
Colour	Pale yellow
Aroma	Conifer
Blends well with	Juniper, Lavender, Sandalwood, Clary Sage, Rosemary, Bergamot, Lemon
Properties	Antirheumatic, Antispasmodic, Hepatic, Sedative

MOST COMMON USES

Emotional	Grief, Insomnia, Danger
Respiratory	Asthma, Coughing, Whooping cough
Skin	Oily, Sweating palms and Feet
Digestive	Diarrhoea, Incontinence
Circulatory	Broken veins, Fluid retention, Varicose veins, Haemorrhoids, Chilblains, Circulation, Cramp
Muscular	Tonic, Rheumatism, Cramp
Gynaecological	Painful periods, Reduces abnormally heavy loss

METHOD OF USE	Bath, Compress, Massage, Vapourizer, Inhaler
CAUTION	Due to possible adulteration

CYPRESS

The common name for this tree is Conifer. This name implies the tree bears cones; a common feature of nearly all the group. The woody cones are made up of tough brown scales usually carrying two seeds. It is important for major suppliers to be aware of the true species being used for oil supply.

The Cypress is a tall vertical evergreen coniferous tree. It has been likened to a finger pointing to the heavens and can reach a height of up to 150ft (45m). The tree bears small flowers and brownish-grey cones. The wood of the Cypress is reddish-yellow, hard yet easy to work; this might be one reason why it was chosen by the Greeks for carving statues of their Gods and by the Phoenicians for building houses and ships.

The Greeks and Romans planted the tree in their cemeteries, probably as a symbol for life after death and possibly because of its evergreen colour or indeed as its name "Sempervirens" suggests " lives forever".

The oil has many uses. I tend to favour it for the following: asthmatic conditions, oedema, heavy periods, varicose veins, piles, oily skin, and in particular sweaty feet.

CYPRESS

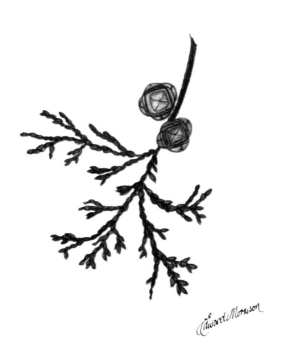

Cupressus Sempervirens

EUCALYPTUS

Note	Top
Botanical Name	Eucalyptus Globulus
Family	Myrtaceae
Cultivation	Spain, Portugal, Australia, Tasmania, Zimbabwe
Part of Plant	Leaves
Extracted by	Steam distillation
Yield 1 Gram Oil	Equals 90 grams base material
Constituents	**Aldehyde** - Citronellal **Oxide**- Cineole **Terpenes** - Camphene, Fenchene, Phellandrene, Pinene
Principal Constituents	Cineole, Pinene
Adulteration	Though a very cheap essential oil it may have synthetic Cineole added or Eucalyptus from various countries.
Colour	Pale yellow
Aroma	Eucalyptus
Blends well with	Benzoin, Lavender, Juniper, Lemongrass, Melissa

| Properties | Antiphlogistic, Antiviral, Bactericide, Decongestant, Stimulant |

MOST COMMON USES

| Emotional | Clears the mind, helps prevent drowsiness |

| Respiratory | Colds, Flu, Throat infections, Sinusitis, Asthma, Bronchitis, Dry cough |

| Skin | Boils, Pimples, Herpes Simplex, Head lice |

| Musculoskeletal | Aches/Pains, Rheumatism, Arthritis |

| Other | Cystitis, Headaches |

| **METHODS OF USE** | Local Massage, Compress, Vaporizer, Local application to skin blemishes, e.g. Boils |

| **CAUTION** | Children - use in very low dilutions. Sensitivity possible in Dermatitis/Eczema skins. |

NOTE !
Death has been reported from oral intake

EUCALYPTUS

Nearly everyone can recognise this oil by its smell (it has a tendency to remind people of illness).

A native of Tasmania and Australia though now cultivated in European countries as well as California and North Africa. The common local name for Eucalyptus is the Gum Tree (due to the sweet smelling gum exuded by the bark). This oil was first distilled in Australia in the 1850's.

The Eucalyptus tree is the tallest deciduous tree on our planet, growing to a height of over 450ft (140-150m). The tree can reach 90ft (27m) in just 20 years. The leaves of the young tree are round and a silvery bluish-green; whereas those of the mature tree are long, pointed and yellowy-green. The oil glands are visible when the leaf is held up to the light. The flowers of the mature tree are a creamy white, the wood is very hard and the bark smooth and pale grey in colour.

My favourite uses for this oil are: - Flu, Bronchitis, Fevers, Shingles and general infections. I use it only in local massage never in a full body treatment.

I always use it in a spray or burner if a member of the household is suffering from any of the above conditions. I also find it useful used in this manner when the usual childhood illnesses are in the family.

As an insect repellent in general Eucalyptus is excellent. Once a month I put a drop of blended oil on my dog's collar to keep them free from little visitors. Used in the same way the oil has a similar benefit for cats.

EUCALYPTUS

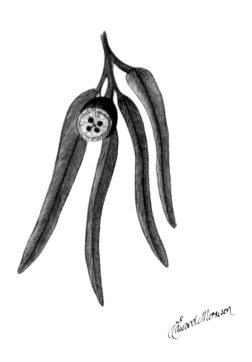

Eucalyptus Globulus

FENNEL SWEET

Note	Middle
Botanical Name	Foeniculum Vulgare
Family	Umbelliferae
Cultivation	Asia (India), USA, Europe (Mediterranean)
Part of Plant	Seed
Extracted by	Steam distillation
Yield 1 Gram Oil	Equals 20 grams base material
Constituents	**Aldehyde** - Cuminic **Ketone** - Fenchone **Terpenes** - Camphene, Dipentene **Phenol -** Anethole, Methylchavicol
Principal Constituents	Anethole, Fenchone
Adulteration	Both with synthetic chemicals and fractions containing components from other essential oils.
Colour	Colourless/pale yellow

Aroma	Warm/aniseed
Blends well with	Geranium, Lavender, Rose, Sandalwood, Rosemary, Lemon
Properties	Antiphlogistic, Antispasmodic, Digestive, Diuretic, Galactagogue

MOST COMMON USES

Digestive	Nausea, Flatulence, Indigestion, Colic, Hiccoughs, Colitis
Gynaecological	Scanty painful periods, PMS.
Other	Cellulite, Urine retention, Urinary tract infection Mouth wash

METHODS OF USE

Bath, Compress, Massage, Mouth wash

CAUTION

Hypersensitive skins. Breastfeeding, Cancer. Anethole may cause allergy.

NOTE !
Maximun 2% blend. This oil is reported to have oestrogenic qualities.

FENNEL

The plant is a native of the Mediterranean although it is now cultivated in many parts of the world. It can grow to about 5 - 6 feet (1.5 - 2 metres) high with feathery blue green leaves and large umbels of yellow flowers about 6 inches (15cms) across, appearing from July to October, followed by greenish yellow or brownish seeds.

The history of Fennel goes back a long way; it was known to the Chinese, Indians, Egyptians, Greeks and Romans. Theophrastus, Pliney, Dioscorides and Hippocrates all mentioned its benefits. The Roman soldiers are said to have carried the seeds on long treks to chew when they were hungry.

Fennel is considered a useful oil for the female reproductive system. Its effects have been known for centuries. It is now thought that this could be due to a hormone, a form of oestrogen, in its structure.

My own main use for the oil is for all the digestive problems, also PMS; scant periods; painful periods; cellulite and fluid retention.

FENNEL

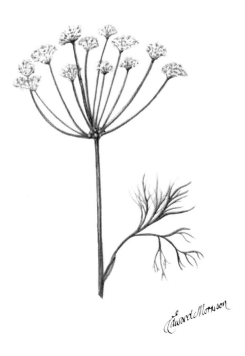

Foeniculum Vulgare

FRANKINCENSE

Note	Middle/Base
Botanical Name	Boswellia Carterii
Family	Burseraceae
Cultivation	Eritrea, India, Aden
Part of Plant	Resin
Extracted by	Steam distillation
Yield 1 Gram Oil	Equals 12 grams base material
Constituents	**Alcohol** - Olibanol **Sesquiterpene** - Cadinene **Terpenes** - Camphene, Dipentene, Pinene, Phellandrene, Thujene
Principal Constituents	Aden Pinene up to 43% Indian Thujene up to 61% Eritrea octyl acetate
Adulteration	Synthetic Pinene added especially to Indian oil which contains very little Pinene.
Colour	Colourless / pale yellow/ yellowish brown
Aroma	Camphorous/Penetrating with a slight hint of lemon

Blends well with	Basil, Black Pepper, Citrus oils, Geranium, Lavender, Sandalwood, Melissa
Properties	Antiseptic, Emollient, Sedative

MOST COMMON USES

Skin	Stretch marks, Mature, Slack, Wrinkled, Inflammation, Boils, Pimples, Scar tissue
Respiratory	Pulmonary antiseptic, Coughs/colds, Bronchial catarrh, Asthma
Emotional	Anxiety
Gynaecological	Heavy periods
Other	Uterine tonic, Gout
METHODS OF USE	Massage, Face creams, Lotions, Local application on skin blemishes
CAUTION	This seems to be a safe oil but like all essential oils needs to be used with care

FRANKINCENSE

Also known as Olibanum, it is a native of the Middle East and Africa. The small tree has abundant pinnate leaves and white to pale pink flowers.

The highly aromatic resin permeates the leaves and bark of the tree and even exudes as a milky juice from the flowers. It is reported that the Bedouins of the past used to visit all the trees in succession and make a deep incision in each, peeling off a narrow strip of bark just below the wound. For the next three months this exercise would be repeated at monthly intervals; each time the original incision would be made deeper.

The large tears are whitish yellow and waxy. They tend to solidify into a yellowish amber colour varying in size from a pea to a walnut. These would be scraped off into large baskets. Every two weeks the harvesters would return to collect the resin until the first rains came and put a close to the year's gatherings.

Frankincense was amongst the most costly substances in the ancient world. It has been used since ancient time in religious rituals and is still used today in incense burners. It was one of the gifts brought to Jesus by the Three Wise Men.

I use the oil in the main for the following conditions: asthma, bronchitis, coughing, heavy periods, mature skin and anxiety.

FRANKINCENSE

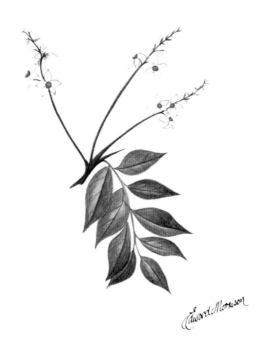

Boswellia Carterii

GERANIUM

Note	Middle
Botanical Name	Pelargonium Graveolens Pelargonium Odorantissimum
Family	Geraniaceae
Cultivation	France, Spain, Italy, Morocco, Egypt (Native Africa)
Part of Plant	Leaves, Flowers
Extracted by	Steam distillation
Yield 1 Gram Oil	Equals 40 grams base material
Constituents	**Acid** - Geranic **Alcohols** - Geraniol, Citronellol, Linalool, Terpineol **Aldehyde** - Citral **Ketone** - Menthone **Phenol** - Eugenol **Terpene** - Sabinene
Principal Constituents	Citronellol, Geraniol
Adulteration	Synthetic considerable due to cost and scarcity of raw material.
Colour	Greenish yellow
Aroma	Graveolens, Rich sweet rose-like Odorantissimum, Slight apple-like

Blends well with	Most oils but especially Lavender, Citrus, Rose, Jasmine, Neroli, Petitgrain
Properties	Adrenal cortex stimulant, Analgesic, Cicatrisant, Diuretic

MOST COMMON USES

Respiratory System	Colds, Flu, Throat / Mouth infections
Skin	Acne, Dry eczema, Herpes Simplex, Stretchmarks, Soothes measles and general rashes
Head	Dandruff, Head lice
Digestive	Diarrhoea, Gastroenteritis
Gynaecological	Hormone imbalance, PMS, Menopausal
Other	Fluid retention, Cellulite, Urinary tract infections, Diabetes
METHODS OF USE	Bath, Compress Massage, Vaporizer, Perfume
CAUTION	Hypersensitive individuals Breast feeding

NOTE !
Reported cases of dermatitis in leaf pickers.

GERANIUM

Pelargonium Graveolens is a perennial plant which grows to about 2-3ft (1m). It has pointed serrated edged leaves and small pink flowers. Although a native of Africa the plant is cultivated in a number of countries. Many species of Pelargonium exist but only about five are used in the production of essential oil. These include Pelargonium Graveolens; Pelargonium Odorantissimum; Pelargonium Capitatum; Pelargonium Roseum (Rose Geranium) and Pelargonium Radula.

Geranium oil is often used to adulterate Rose oil. Geranium itself is quite expensive, so once again be warned that there are no bargains in essential oil quality. The most expensive oil comes from the Reunion, an island in the South West Indian ocean.

The 19th century saw the first distillation of essential oils from France. There is not a lot of information about Geranium in the history books until Culpepper's Herbal was published in 1653; although mention had previously been made by Dioscorides about a "Geranion". However, we are unsure if this was reference to the same plant (Geranium).

Geranium is reported to be an adrenal cortex stimulant. I find Geranium to be a most useful oil and use it for the following conditions: Menopausal symptoms, PMS, fluid retention, cellulite, depression, all skin types (as a balancer), insect repellent and air freshener/deodoriser.

NOTE !
If used at night on those who normally cannot sleep it may not be helpful unless blended in a low percentage and used with a sedative oil.

GERANIUM

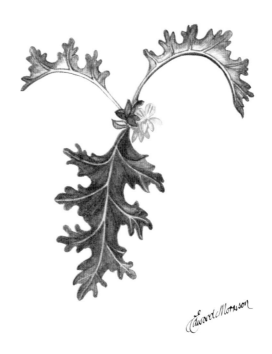

Pelargonium Graveolens

GINGER

Note	Base
Botanical Name	Zingiber Officinale
Family	Zingiberaceae
Cultivation	India, China
Part of Plant	Roots
Extracted by	Distillation
Yield 1 Gram Oil	Equals 40 grams base material
Constituents	**Alcohol** - Borneol **Aldehyde** - Citral **Oxide** - Cineole **Sesquiterpene** - Zingiberene **Terpenes** - Camphene, Limonene, Phellandrene
Principal Constituents	Zingiberene, Cineole
Adulteration	Rarely, however, Galanga oil can be used for this purpose. Main differences occur in the composition of oil from different countries.
Colour	Pale greenish yellow/ deep yellow
Aroma	Fresh root ginger/sweet/ woody
Blends well with	Citrus, Eucalyptus, Frankinscence, Geranium, Rosemary

| Properties | Analgesic, Antiemetic, Rubefacient, Stomachic, |

MOST COMMON USES

Musculoskeletal	Rheumatic pain, Muscular pain, Arthritis
Respiratory	Catarrh, Colds, Flu, Sore Throats
Digestive	Diarrhoea, Travel sickness

| **METHODS OF USE** | Compress, Local massage, Vaporizer |

| **CAUTION** | Minor phototoxic effects though this will be enhanced if Ginger oil is used together with other phototoxic oils. May cause skin reaction in hypersensitive individuals. |

GINGER

A perennial plant with reedlike leaves and thick rhizomes which are tubelike and knotted on both sides.

Ginger was mentioned in old Chinese manuscripts. It was also known to the Greeks and Romans but was not discovered in Europe until the middle ages.

Ginger contains about 2% volatile oil. It is sensitive to strong sunlight and so is grown in the shade of other crops.

When the stems dry off the tubers are ready for harvesting.

The most common use I have for this oil is for treating localised areas of muscular type pain and for digestive disorders.

GINGER

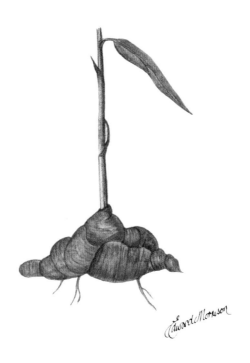

Zingiber Officinale

GRAPEFRUIT

Note	Top
Botanical Name	Citrus Paradisi
Family	Rutaceae
Cultivation	USA, South Africa
Part of Plant	Rind of fruit
Extracted by	Expression
Yield 1 Gram Oil	Equals 250 grams base material
Constituents	**Alcohols** - Geraniol, Linalool **Aldehyde** - Citral **Terpenes** - Limonene, Pinene
Principal Constituents	Limonene
Adulteration	With inferior oil from fruit once the juice is extracted.
Colour	Yellow/greenish

Aroma	Tangy
Blends well with	Most other oils
Properties	Antidepressant, Digestive, Stimulant, Tonic

MOST COMMON USES

Emotional	Mental stimulant
Digestive	Indigestion, Liver and Gallbladder problems

METHODS OF USE	Bath, Massage, Compress
CAUTION	Slight phototoxicity. Short shelf life.

GRAPEFRUIT

The Grapefruit grows on a fairly tall sturdy tree approximately 18ft (6m) tall with dense foliage of dark green, glossy leaves. The large white flowers are borne single or in clusters in the axils of the leaves. Mature trees produce large crops of the fruit, (up to 1500lbs per tree).

The fruit which is yellow when ripe, ranges from 4-6 inches (100-150mm) in diameter, twice the size of the average orange. It became a well established fruit in the islands of the West Indies before coming to the mainland USA. Other producing countries include Israel, Brazil and South Africa.

The essential oil is best when expressed. A slightly inferior oil is distilled.

I tend to reach for the grapefruit oil most often when treating people with stress related problems. I find also that the Grapefruit added to a floral oil helps to give the aroma a more sharp but pleasing smell.

I do not use this oil if the skin shows signs of Melanoma, Pre-Melanoma, large dark moles or any skin Cancers.

GRAPEFRUIT

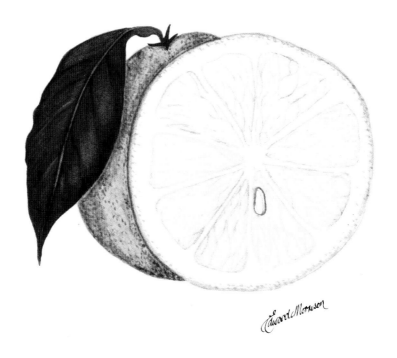

Citrus Paradisi

JASMINE

Note	Middle/Base
Botanical Name	Jasminum Officinale or Jasminum Grandiflorum
Family	Oleaceae
Cultivation	France, Algeria, Egypt, Morocco, China
Part of Plant	Flowers
Extracted by	Enfleurage, Solvent extraction
Yield 1 Gram Oil	Equals 900 grams base material
Constituents	**Alcohols** - Benzyl alcohol, Farnesol, Geraniol, Nerol, Terpineol, Linalool **Esters** - Benzyl acetate, Methyl anthranilate **Ketone** - Jasmone **Phenol** - Eugenol
Principal Constituents	Benzyl acetate, Linalool Over 100 constituents in this oil
Adulteration	Due to high cost of true Jasmine the oil is often adulterated with synthetic components and or Ylang-Ylang oil components.

Colour	Reddish brown
Aroma	Floral/ sweet/ slightly heady
Blends well with	All oils but especially Citrus
Properties	Antidepressant, Parturient, Sedative, Uterine

MOST COMMON USES

Emotional	Depression, Tension, Anxiety, Confidence
Gynaecological	Menstrual pain/cramp, Labour pains
Other	Male prostate gland, Dry skin, Dry coughs
METHODS OF USE	Bath, Compress, Massage, Vapouriser, Perfume
CAUTIONS	Use in low dilutions ½ to 1½%. May cause allergic reaction in hypersensitive individuals.

NOTE !
Considered a useful oil during labour.

JASMINE

The common name of Jasmine is used for the genus Jasminum of the Oleaceae family (Olive family). Personally I prefer this fragrance to all others.

A vine-like deciduous shrub which grows to over 30ft high it has long smooth, slender branches with oval pointed leaves.
The pinwheel shaped white flower head grows on a thin pedicel and opens at night. This night opening is the reason the flowers have to be picked at night, at this time the odour is at its most powerful.

The plant originates from Iran and India although it is now grown in Egypt, Morocco, Italy and France. France is now a major producer.

Jasmine is one of the most expensive oils to purchase, however only a very small amount is necessary, as low as 1 drop in 10ml or even 20ml of base oil.

Jasmine is classified amongst the aphrodisiacs and is important to the perfumery industry as no synthetic equivalent has been created. The oil is used in Femme by Rochas, Chanel No 5 and Samsara by Guerlain. Some perfume houses have resorted to buying their own Jasmine fields.

I use it mainly for the following conditions : Scant periods, PMS, nervousness, lack of self esteem, frigidity and as a confidence booster.

JASMINE

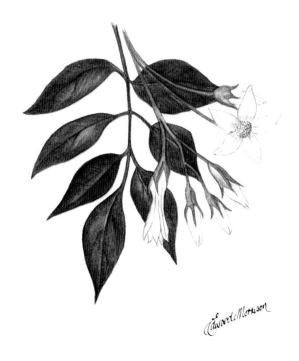

Jasminum Officinale

JUNIPER

Note	Middle
Botanical Name	Juniperus Communis
Family	Cupressaceae
Cultivation	Yugoslavia, Italy, France
Part of Plant	Ripe berries
Extracted by	Steam distillation
Yield 1 Gram Oil	Equals 100 grams base material
Constituents	**Alcohols** - Borneol, Terpineol **Sesquiterpenes** - Cadinene, Cedrene **Terpenes** - Camphene, Myrcene, Pinene, Sabinene
Principal Constituents	Myrcene, Pinene
Adulteration	Juniper twig oil and juniper wood oil can be added. Also or instead fractions of turpentine oil and synthetic components may be added.
Colour	Colourless/pale greenish-yellow

Aroma	Slight turpentine, Balsmic, Hot, Woody
Blends well with	Rosemary, Cypress, Lavender, Sandalwood, Geranium, Bergamot, Frankincense
Properties	Antirheumatic, Diuretic, Stimulating

MOST COMMON USES

Musculoskeletal	Aches, Pain, Rheumatism
Digestive	Indigestion, Flatulence, Diarrhoea, Colic
Emotional	Anxiety/Stress
Skin	Acne, Oily, Congested, Seborrhoea of scalp
Other	Scanty periods, Fluid retention

METHODS OF USE	Massage, Vaporiser
CAUTION	Kidney conditions. Oil reported to be Nephrotoxic and may also be a slight skin irritant on those prone to sensitivity.

JUNIPER

An evergreen shrub found in dry soil it usually grows to a height of 12ft (2 - 4m) though has been known to grow as tall as 25ft (over 7m). The bark is a dark brown tinged with red. A pretty coloured shrub, Juniper's needle-shaped leaves have white stripes on top and shiny yellow/ green underneath. On the male tree the flowers are yellow.

Flowering time is April to June. The berry fruit is green in the first year ripening to a blue black with a grey tinge in the second.

Reference to Juniper was made by the Egyptians and Greeks.
The Romans used it as an antiseptic; Galan and Pliny mentioned its use for liver complaints and St. Hildegard prescribed it for pulmonary infections. Herbalists throughout the ages have mentioned the virtues of Juniper.

I find this oil most useful when treating congested, spotty skin especially on the back, (blended with Tea-Tree). Also for sluggish circulation and cellulite, (provided no kidney disorders).

JUNIPER

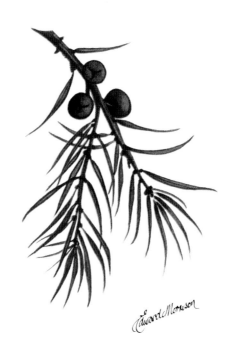

Juniperus Communis

LAVENDER

Note	Middle/Base
Botanical Name	Lavendula Officinalis Lavendula Angustifolia
Family	Labiatae
Cultivation	France, England, Spain and the former USSR
Part of Plant	Flowers
Extracted by	Steam distillation
Yield 1 Gram Oil	Equals 145 grams base material
Constituents	**Alcohols** - Borneol, Geraniol, Lavandulol,Linalool **Ester** - Geranyl acetate, Lavandulol acetate, Linalyl acetate **Oxide** -Cineole **Sesquiterpene** - Caryophyllene **Terpenes** - Limonene, Pinene
Principal Constituents	Limonene, Linal acetate, Linalool
Adulteration	Lavindin (due to cheapness). Fractions of Rosewood and Ho-leaf due to Linalool and
Linalyl	acetate content.
Colour	Pale yellow/ yellowish-green

Aroma	Classical/ mossy/woody
Blends well with	Most oils, Citrus, Clary Sage, Bergamot, Geranium, Patchouli, Rosemary; though less well with the exotic such as Ylang-Ylang, Jasmine, etc.
Properties	Antidepressant, Antispasmodic, Antiviral, Antiseptic
MOST COMMON USES	Burns, Bites, Lice, Stings, Anxiety, Nervous tension, Immune, Deficiency, Insomnia, Eczema, Dermatitis
METHODS OF USE	Bath, Compress, Massage, Inhaler, Vapouriser
CAUTION	If adulteration has occured phototoxic caution should be exercised.

NOTE !
Considered suitable for childeren and frail individuals. Like all essential oil it is not recommended for use on children under one year old.

LAVENDER

The most commonly used essential oil

LAVENDER

A fragrant spreading shrub with grey-green, narrow, linear, downy leaves and purple-blue flowers that are borne on long slender stems. The plant reaches a height of about 3ft (1m).

The Lavender originates from the Mediterranean although it is now cultivated in most parts of the world including Norfolk U.K. Lavender from the famous Grasse area of France is prized for its strong sweet fragrance. The English Lavender has a slightly more camphoric smell. In the 1700's the Lavender fields of Mitcham, Surrey were harvested by the perfumers Yardley.

Before the invention of modern machinery the farmers of old would climb the mountains in the scorching midday sun to cut the Lavender, tie it into bundles and carry it on their backs down the mountainside to the village still, where all the varieties of Lavender were distilled together. Today this work is done mainly by machines harvesting the lavender from Lavender fields; with the Lavenders being classified and distilled separately.

The whole plant is highly aromatic. The best quality oil is produced from the flowers though some oil is produced from the stalk and the leaves.

Lavender like a lot of our Aromatherapy oils, has a long history, being mentioned by Dioscorides, Galen, Pliny and St. Hildegard. The Romans used it on their wounds and added it to their bath water. It was popular in the Elizabethan, Stuart and even Victorian times, also Lavender sachets were sewn into dresses and skirt hems and placed in linen cupboards. Dr. Jean Valnet, an army surgeon, used the oils to treat the war wounded.

In more modern times Lavender was made famous by the French chemist Dr. Renée Gattefosse when he severely burned his hand in the laboratory and plunged it into the nearest bowl of liquid; it transpired that the bowl contained Lavender oil. The pain eased and the burn healed very quickly. It is Dr. Renée Gattefosse who coined the word Aromatherapy.

Every household should have a bottle of Lavender in the First Aid Box. It is the most versatile and most commonly used of all oils with an odour that is second in popularity only to that of Rose or Jasmine and it blends well with almost all other oils.

Lavender is one of the few oils that can be applied neat to the skin. If treating a burn use neat oil, not blended, then cover the area with a cold damp gauze or hankie, (not cotton wool). Normal treatment for a burn is to plunge the burn into ice cold water or put under a cold running tap until pain eases. If Lavender oil is available use next.

I use Lavender in the main to treat the following conditions: acne, burns, bites, stings, bruises, cuts, grazes, cystitis, leucorrhoea, rheumatic conditions, gout, colds, flu, cold sores, shingles, insomnia, migraine, (childhood illnesses, very low dilutions, as little as ¼% up to 1% depending on age) and as an insect repellent.

All childhood illnesses should be medically investigated.

Serious burns need medical attention.

LAVENDER

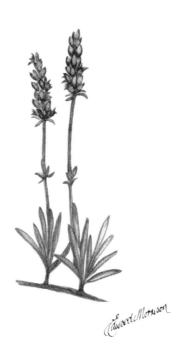

Lavendula Officinalis

LEMON

Note	Top
Botanical Name	Citrus Limonum
Family	Rutaceae
Cultivation	India, Israel, Italy, Spain, France, (Mediterranean), USA
Part of Plant	Fruit peel
Extracted by	Expression
Yield 1 Gram Oil	Equals 200 grams base material
Constituents	**Alcohol** - Linalool **Aldehydes** - Citral, Citronellal **Sesquiterpenes** - Bisabolene, Cadinene **Terpenes** - Camphene, Dipentene, Limonene, Pinene, Phellandrene
Principal Constituents	Limonene. Minor component: Furacumarines - Bergaptene.
Adulteration	Common and difficult to detect; cheap Orange and or Citral from Lemongrass, Synthetic Limonene. Antioxidants (to prevent oxidation) to prolong shelf life.
Colour	Pale yellow/yellowish green

Aroma	Lemon
Blends well with	Lavender, Neroli and all the floral and exotic oils
Properties	Antineuralgic, Astringent, Bactericide

MOST COMMON USES

Respiratory	Throat infections, Colds and Flu
Skin	Greasy, Herpes simplex, Wounds, Boils, Spots, Brightens dull discoloured skins
Musculoskeletal	Arthritis, Rheumatism
Digestive	Heartburn, Gastric acidity, Indigestion, Liver
Circulation	High blood pressure, Varicose veins, Sluggish circulation
Other	Cellulite, Fluid retention, Haemorrhoids, Diabetes. Household antiseptic Mouth wash
METHODS OF USE	Compress, Local massage, Vapouriser
CAUTION	Phototoxicity depends on actual components of the oil varying from high to low. Assume high until proven otherwise. The oil might cause irritation on eczema / dermatitis type skin.

LEMON

The Lemon is a small thorny evergreen that grows up to about 16ft (5m) high.

The Lemon Tree originated in China, India and Japan but is now cultivated in the USA and in many Mediterranean countries especially Italy, Spain, France, Sicily and Cyprus.

The leaves of the Lemon tree are egg-shaped and slightly scalloped. The white flowers appear singularly or in pairs. The fruit of this tree is too well known to warrant description.

The oil was used in French hospitals as a disinfectant up to the First World War. Most people like the fragrance of Lemon oil.

I find that I use this oil most for the following :- Sweaty feet, air disinfectant, varicose veins, insect bites, bronchitis, laryngitis, diabetes, hand and nail treatments.

I do not use this oil if the skin shows signs of Melanoma, Pre-Melanoma, large dark moles or any skin Cancers

LEMON

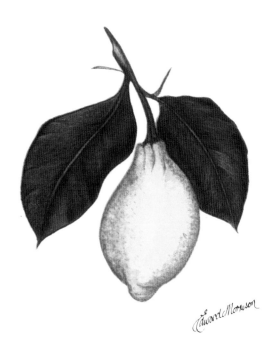

Citrus Limonum

LEMONGRASS

Note	Top
Botanical Name	Cymbopogan Citratus
Family	Gramineae
Cultivation	Brazil, Central Africa, Malay, Madras
Part of Plant	Leaves
Extracted by	Steam distillation
Yield 1 Gram Oil	Equals 15 grams base material
Constituents	**Alcohols** - Farnesol, Geraniol, Nerol **Aldehydes** - Citral Citronellal **Terpenes** - Limonene, Myrcene
Principal Constituents	Citral, Limonene
Adulteration	Unlikely as the oil is very cheap
Colour	Yellow/golden, reddish brown
Aroma	Fresh, lemony
Blends well with	Geranium, Jasmine, Lavender, Rosemary, Rose, Neroli, Tea-Tree

Properties	Antiseptic, Bactericide, Fungicide, Insecticide

MOST COMMON USES Feverish conditions, Infectious diseases, Gastroenteritis, Colitis, Fungal infections

Other Insect repellent, Household antiseptic

METHODS OF USE Local massage, Foot bath, Vaporiser

CAUTION Might cause dermal irritation in susceptable individuals.
Do not use on small children, breast feeding mothers or on people who suffer with glaucoma.
High doses of Citral may cause rise in occular tension.

NOTE !
Citral from Lemongrass is used for the production of vitamin A.

LEMONGRASS

A fragrant tropical grass which grows up to 3ft (1m) high. It reproduces by root division.

A native of Asia now cultivated in India, Sri Lanka, Indonesia and Africa as well as North and South America. The Lemongrass is a member of the family of tropical grasses like Palmarosa, Vetiver and Citronella.

Between two and three crops of grass are cut each year. This tends to exhaust a soil that is not properly fertilised and means that the grasses have to be moved to new ground every few years in order to sustain the quality.

I personally use this oil for tired, aching muscles especially after long journeys sitting down. I use it also as an insect repellent.

LEMONGRASS

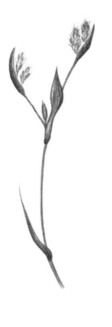

Cymbopogan Citratus

LIME

Note	Top
Botanical Name	Citrus Aurantifolia
Family	Rutaceae
Cultivation	Italy, USA
Part of Plant	Rind of Fruit
Extracted by	Expression Steam distillation (Crushed fruit)
Yield 1 Gram oil	Equals 220 grams base material
Constituents	**Alcohol** - Linalool **Aldehyde** - Citral **Oxide** - Cineole **Terpenenes** - Limonene, Pinene Camphene, Sabinene
Principal Constituants	Limonene, Pinene **Expressed** Oil from peel contains phototoxic chemicals including Bergaptene **Distilled** Oil from whole fruit does not contain phototoxic chemicals
Adulteration	Other lime species, distilled / expressed oils mixed together.

Colour	Pale yellow/yellowish green
Aroma	Sharp citrus
Blends well with	Florals and citrus oils
Properties	Antiseptic, Antineuralgic, Astingent, Bactericide, Carminative

MOST COMMON USES

Skin	Boils, Spots, Herpes Simplex
Curculation	Sluggish circulation, Varicose veins
Respiration	Colds, Sore throats
Musculoskeletal	Joint aches/pains

METHODS OF USE	Compress, Massage
CAUTION	Unless sure of quality and extraction method, treat as phototoxic. Avoid exposure to UV (sunbed/sun) for 12 hours prior to or after use of Lime oil.

NOTE !
Lime juice is used to produce citric acid.

LIME

A small evergreen tree that grows about 4-5m high, the leaves are oval and the flowers small and white.

The tree probably originated in Asia though it is now found in the USA and many Mediterranean countries especially Italy. Limes were brought to the USA from Spain and Portugal around the 16th century. Ships carrying the limes were called Lime Juicers since the crews ate the limes and drank the juice to prevent scurvy.

The essential oil is similar to Lemon in so far as the distilled version of the oil comes from crushed fruit. Lime is used extensively in the perfumery industry.

I love the fresh smell of lime oil. I use it mainly for skins that are a little oily especially if there are a few spots, I also find it useful on general grazes obtained on a sports field.

When used with strong floral smelling oils it gives a nice sharpness to the blend, making the floral more acceptable to the male senses.

NOTE !
I have known lime oil to cause allergic reaction in two people who were known hay fever sufferers.

LIME

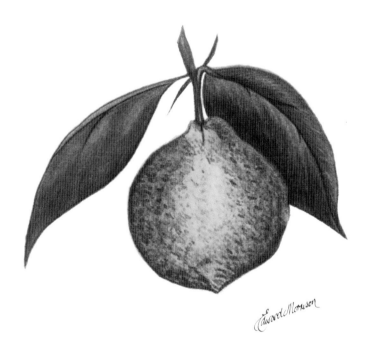

Citrus Aurantifolia

MANDARIN

Note	Top
Botanical Name	Citrus Madurensis
Family	Rutaceae
Cultivation	Brazil,Spain,Italy, California.
Part of Plant	Peel
Extracted by	Expression
Yield 1 Gram Oil	Equals 150 grams of base material
Constituents	**Alcohol** - Geraniol **Aldehydes** - Citral Citronellal **Ester** - Methyl acetate **Terpene** - Limonene
Principal Constituants	Limonene, Geraniol
Adulteration	With other species plus Tangerine and may have cheap orange added.
Colour	Golden with a faint blue tint which becomes visible in bright light.

Properties	Antispasmodic, Digestive, Sedative, Tonic

MOST COMMON USES — Depression, Anxiety, Stress, Flatulence, Irritability
PMS, Stimulates appetite, Stimulates liver, Stretch marks, Scarring

Other — Insomnia
Rich in vitamin C
Perfume

METHODS OF USE — Bath, Compress, Massage, Vaporiser

CAUTION — Avoid exposure to sun/sunbed for twelve hours prior to or after use of oil and be especially careful if oil is adulterated.

NOTE !
Considered useful for children and the elderly, also acne type skins.

MANDARIN

A native of China and the Far East, Mandarin was brought to Europe at the beginning of the 19th century. It is an evergreen with small glossy leaves and fragrant flowers. The tree grows to about 20ft (6m) in height and bears a very sweet yellowy fruit which contains pips.

My main use for Mandarin is to blend with the heavy floral oils to give a more pleasing smell and also to treat general digestive and liver problems. I will, on occasion, use this oil to treat skin recovering from acne.

I do not use this oil if the skin shows signs of Melanoma, Pre-Melanoma, large dark moles or any skin Cancers.

MANDERIN

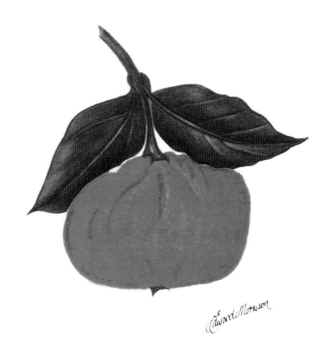

Citrus Madurensis

MARJORAM

Note	Middle
Botanical Name	Origanum Marjorana
Family	Labiatae
Cultivation	Spain, France, Tunisia
Part of Plant	Flowering tops/leaves
Extracted by	Steam distillation
Yield 1 Gram Oil	Equals 200 grams base material
Constituents	**Alcohols** -Borneol,Terpineol **Ketone** -Camphor **Sesquiterpene** -Caryophyllene **Terpenes** - Pinene, Sabinene, Terpinene
Principal Constituants	Terpinene, Terpineol
Adulteration	Substitution Spanish for French. Mixing Thyme, Tea Tree, Oreganum, Terpenes from other oils.
Colour	Yellowish/dark brown
Aroma	Spicy/ slightly peppery
Blends well with	Bergamot, Lemon, Lavender, Rosemary, Rosewood, Ylang-Ylang

Properties	Analgesic, Carminative, Cephalic, Hypotensive

MOST COMMON USES

Emotional	Anxiety, Tension, Hysteria, Loneliness, Grief, Insomnia
Respiratory	Asthma, Colds, Bronchitis
Vascular	High Blood Pressure (dilates arteries)
Musculoskeletal	Cramps, Aches and Pains,Sprains and Strains, Rheumatism, Arthritis
Neurological	Neuralgia
Digestive	Colic, Constipation, Indigestion, Flatulence
Gynaecological	Menstrual cramp, Period pain
METHODS OF USE	Bath, Compress, Massage, Vapouriser, Inhaler
CAUTION	Strong sedative effect and overuse may have stupefying effect. Reported as unsuitable for use with low blood pressure.

NOTE !
Considered a useful oil for treating individuals who suffer with high blood pressure.

MARJORAM

The plant known as Sweet or Knotted Marjoram is a small shrub which can grow to a height of about 20 inches (50cm). It is native to the Mediterranean although it is cultivated widely.

The stems, red to brownish red, are mainly upright and stout. The flowers are small, white or pink in colour and arranged in small rounded spikes. Flowering time is midsummer to early Autumn.

St. Hildegarde thought it a cure for leprosy. Dioscorides recommended it for animal bites, the Romans used it to drive away ants and the Greeks used it to treat spasm (Theophrastus mentioned it as a medicinal plant). During the Middle Ages it was used not only in a medicinal role but also in superstition. Nearer to present time, in the 1600's, nosegays contained Marjoram to mask unpleasant smells.

The oil has a strong smell which is acceptable to both males and females and is considered an anaphrodisiac. This is brought about not by hormonal reaction but by the oil's lessening effects on the emotional level.

My uses for this oil are many but in particular for high blood pressure, heart conditions, asthma, menstrual cramp, intestinal cramp, rheumatism, arthritis, insomnia, and on aching/painful muscles after exercise.

MARJORAM

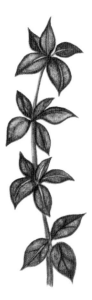

Origanum Marjorana

MELISSA

Note	Middle
Botanical Name	Melissa Officinalis
Family	Labiatae
Cultivation	France, (Mediterranean) USA
Part of Plant	Leaves/Flowers
Extracted by	Steam distillation
Yield 1 Gram Oil	Equals 900 grams base material
Constituents	**Acid** - Citronellic **Alcohols** - Citronellol, Geraniol, Linalool **Aldehydes** - Citral, Citronellal **Ester** - Geranyl acetate **Sesquiterpene** - Caryophyllene
Principal Constituants	Geranial Acetate, Caryophyllene, Citronellal
Adulteration	Due to low yield and high cost, most Melissa oil is adulterated with synthetic chemicals. May be mixed with Lemon, Lemongrass or Verbena oil amongst others.
Colour	Very pale brownish

Aroma	Fresh lemony
Blends well with	Geranium, Lavender, Neroli, Ylang-Ylang, Jasmine, Rose, Rosemary, Chamomile
Properties	Antidepressant, Carminative, Hypotensive, Nervine

MOST COMMON USES

Emotional	Depression, Insomnia, Migraine, Anxiety, Emotional shock, Grief, Shingles, Cold sores
Other	Flatulence High blood pressure

METHODS OF USE	Bath, Compress, Massage, Vapouriser
CAUTION	Not to be used on damaged or diseased skin or for children under the age of three. Glaucoma, Breast feeding.

NOTE !
True Melissa contains chemicals that have anti-viral properties, however it is believed that most are lost during steam distillation.

MELISSA

A native of Southern Europe this strong perennial has small green slightly hairy, wrinkled leaves, tiny yellowish white flowers and grows to about 2ft (60cms) tall. During May and June the plant is harvested prior to the flower opening.

The name is derived from the Latin name for honey. Bees seem to love the Melissa plant. Theophrastus and Dioscorides wrote about the "bee plant". In the 14th century a group of French Carmelite nuns produced a tonic water containing Melissa.

I would suggest that this oil is used only by the more experienced therapist who is absolutely sure of the origin and purity of the oil.

I use the oil most often when treating the following conditions: shock, bereavement, asthma, high blood pressure or irregular periods.

Today I question the quality of Melissa and wonder if I am really getting value for money and passing on value for money.
I am now considering removing this oil from my collection.

MELISSA

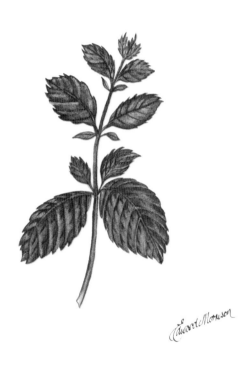

Melissa Officinalis

MYRRH

Note	Base
Botanical Name	Commiphora myrrha
Family	Burseraceae
Cultivation	North Eastern Africa, Libya
Part of Plant	Resin from trunk
Extracted by	Steam distillation
Yield 1 Gram Oil	Equals 15 grams base material
Constituents	**Acids** - Myrrholic **Aldehydes** - Cinnamic, Cuminic **Sesquiterpenes** - Cadinene **Phenols** - Eugenol **Terpenes** - Dipentene, Limonene, Heerabolene, Pinene
Principal Constituants	Heerabolene, Limonene, Eugenol
Adulteration	Myrrh absolute decolourised and referred to as essential oil. Essential oil mixed with Opoponax (Hercules Auheel).
Colour	Pale yellow

Aroma	Musty/ incense-like
Blends well with	Camphor, Lavender
Properties	Astringent, Anti-inflammatory, Expectorant, Fungicidal,

MOST COMMON USES

Skin	Slow healing wounds, Eczema, Athlete's foot, Chapped skin, Mouth ulcers, Gum disorders
Respiratory	Chest infections, Catarrh, Chronic bronchitis, Colds, Sore throats
Digestive	Diarrhoea, Flatulence, Tonic
Other	Thrush, Haemorrhoids, Loss of appetite
METHODS OF USE	Bath, Local massage
CAUTION	Possibly toxic in high concentrations.

MYRRH

A good sized bushy tree growing to about 9ft (3m). The trifoliate leaves are scanty and aromatic growing on sturdy knotted branches. The flowers are small and white.

Myrrh was first recognised in the early 19th century in a place known as Ghizan on the Red Sea coast, an area so dry and barren that it is called Tehama meaning "Hell".

The Myrrh bush has natural ducts in the bark. The tissue between the ducts breaks down forming cavities these cavities become filled with a granular secretion. When, either through natural fissures or through incision the bark is broken a thick pale yellow liquid flows out. This liquid hardens to a reddish-brown colour forming brittle tears known as Myrrh.

My main use for this oil is in the treatment of slow healing wounds such as ulcers. I have also found it useful for boils when blended with Lavender or Tea-Tree. I have used it with some success on chapped skin brought on by weather conditions.

MYRRH

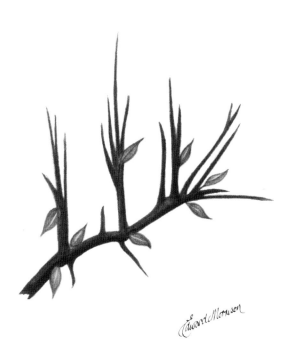

Commiphora myrrha

NEROLI

Note	Middle/Base
Botanical Name	Citrus Aurantium/Vulgaris
Family	Rutaceae
Cultivation	France, Tunisia
Part of Plant	Flowers
Extracted by	Enfieurage/ Steam distillation
Yield 1 Gram Oil	Equals 1000 grams base material
Constituents	**Acid** - Phenylacetic **Alcohols** - Nerol, Geraniol, Linalool, Nerolodol,Terpineol **Esters** - Linalyl acetate, Methyl anthranilate, Neryl acetate **Ketone** - Jasmone **Nitrogen** -Indole **Terpenes** - Camphene, Limonene
Principal Constituents	Linal acetate, Linalool, Geraniol
Adulteration	Very common due to high cost of the oil. Substitutions Petitgrain, Bitter Orange Oil, also Synthetic Linal acetate and or Linalool amongst other additions.
Colour	Pale yellow

Aroma	Sweet/ floral but somewhat seaweed-like
Blends well with	Most oils especially Bergamot, Lemon, Lavender, Rosemary, Sandalwood, Clary-Sage, Jasmine and Rose
Properties	Antidepressant, Aphrodisiac, Cytophylactic, Sedative

MOST COMMON USES

Emotional	Anxiety, Depression, Stress, Shock, Overwork, Insomnia, Bereavement
Skin	All skin types, especially mature, dry and sensitive
Digestive	Chronic diarrhoea, Intestinal spasm, Flatulence
Other	Palpitations, Panic
METHODS OF USE	Bath, Massage, Inhaler, Vaporizer, Perfume
CAUTION	Reported to cause drowsiness if overused.

NEROLI

Neroli is extracted from the white petals of the Bitter or Seville Orange Tree which grows up to a height of 30ft (9m). The tree originated in China but is now found throughout the Mediterranean. The best and most expensive oil comes from France, Tunisia and Sicily. It is a pale yellow liquid which darkens on exposure to light.

Neroli was first discovered in the mid 17th century and is thought to have been named after an Italian princess, Ann Marie who lived in Neroli (near Rome). She used the oil as her favourite perfume and to scent her gloves and her bath water.

Orange flowers are worn in wedding bouquets and bridal head dresses as a symbol of love and innocence; however this has not always been so. It is said that the perfume was once worn by prostitutes so that their customers could recognise them by their smell.

Neroli is a very useful oil, although to smell it in its pure state I think it can be off putting and strong. When blended however, it has a most beautiful smell and is without doubt one of my own favourites.

It has many uses in Aromatherapy. I tend to use it for the following conditions: acne, anxiety, insomnia, skin care (all types), shock, nervous tummies (especially if spasm or diarrhoea present).

Neroli is a very relaxing oil and a reputed aphrodisiac.

NEROLI

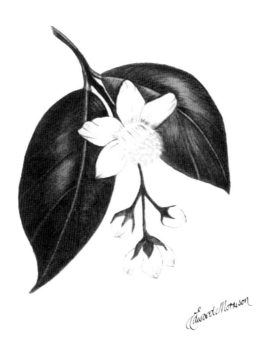

Citrus Aurantium/Vulgaris

NIAOULI

Note	Top
Botanical Name	Melaleuca Viridiflora
Family	Myrtaceae
Cultivation	Australia, Tasmania, New Caledonia
Part of Plant	Leaves, Young twigs
Extracted by	Distillation
Yeild 1 Gram Oil	Equals 100 grams of base material
Constituents	**Acid** - Valeric **Alcohol** - Terpineol **Keytone** - Cineole **Terpenes** - Liomonen, Pinene
Principal Constituants	Cineole
Adulteration	When this takes place it is with Cajuput and / or Eucalyptus.
Colour	Colourless/ Pale yellow/green
Aroma	Clear sweet Camphoraceous
Blends well with	Citrus, Fennel, Juniper, Peppermint, Pine, Rosemary and Lavender

Properties	Analgesic, Antiseptic, Antispasmodic, Bactericide, Expectorant, Insecticide, Balsamic, Cicartrisant

MOST COMMON USES

Skin	Acne, Boils, Spots, Ulcers, Cuts, Insect bites
Respiratory	Brochitis, Coughs, Sinusitis, Catarrhal conditions
Urinary	Cystitis, Urinary infections
Muscles	Aches, Pains
Immune System	Fevers, Flu / colds
METHODS OF USE	Bath, Inhalation, Massage, Vaporiser, Spray
CAUTION	None apparent

NOTE !
A non toxic oil. Take care to ensure quality as it may be adulterated.

NIAOULI

A large evergreen tree with a flexible trunk that grows abundantly in Australia, the foliage is bushy with pointed leaves and yellow flowers. When crushed the leaves give off strong scent. Niaouli is a member of the Tea-Tree family. The oil is similar to Cajeput and sometimes used as a substitute for Cajeput and or Eucalyptus.

The plant was assigned its botanical name during Captain Cook's voyage to Australia in 1788.

The oil is sometimes referred to by the French term Gomenol, a name derived from the fact it was once shipped from Gomen in the French East Indies.

Niaouli was once added to beverages and drunk in the Middle East. It was used locally to purify the water as well as for aches, pains and all sorts of infections. In France it was used as an antiseptic in the obstetric units.

I use Niaouli for general cases where the immune system is weak, also for oily/spotty skins. I find its aroma is well tolerated by male clients.

NIAOULI

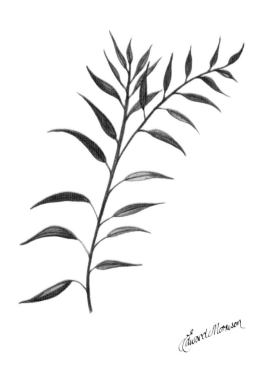

Melaleuca Viridiflora

PALMAROSA

Note	Top
Botanical Name	Cymbopogon Martini
Family	Gramineae
Cultivation	India, Pakistan, Africa and Indonesia
Part of Plant	Dried grass
Extracted by	Steam distillation
Yeild 1 Gram Oil	Equals 70 grams of base material
Constituents	**Alcohol** - Geraniol, Citronellol, Farnesol **Aldehyde** - Citral, Citronellal **Ester** - Geranyl acetate **Terpenes** - Limonene, Dipentene
Principal Constituents	Geraniol
Adulteration	Gingergrass, Turpentine, Citronella or synthetic Geraniol may be added.
Colour	Pale yellow/ Orange

Aroma	Sweet/ Rosy geranium-like
Blends well with	Florals and woods
Properties	Antiseptic, Antiviral, Bactericide, Febrifuge, Hydrating, Stimulant (Digestive, Circulation)

MOST COMMON USES

Skin	All skin types, (balancing) Dermatitis, Acne
Digestive	Infections, Anorexia (appetite stimulant)
Nervous	Stress, Nervous exhaustion.
Immune	Fevers
METHODS OF USE	Bath, Massage, Spray, Perfume
CAUTION	None apparent

NOTE!
Commonly known as Turkish Geranium and East Indian Geranium.

PALMAROSA

A wild growing, spreading, grass like plant with long, slender stems. The grass is harvested before the flowering tops appear and the largest yield is obtained when the grass is allowed to dry, which takes about a week from cutting.

Palmarosa has been known as Indian Geranium and Turkish Geranium. The names date back to the time when the oil was shipped from Bombay to ports of the Red Sea and then transported partly by land to Constantinople and Bulgaria where the oil was often used to adulterate Rose oil.

Gingergrass is sometimes sold as Palmarosa but although closely related Gingergrass is of inferior quality containing less geraniol. Natives evaluate the quality of the oil by hitting the bottle of oil against the palm of the hand and if the air bubbles rising to the surface disappear quickly then the oil is assumed to be of good quality.

I find this a very useful oil to have in my selection, especially for facial treatment and have found it to be a favourite with those clients who have eating disorders.

PALMAROSA

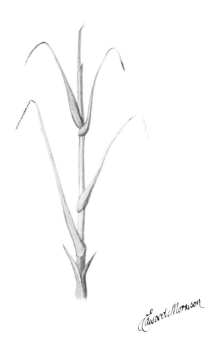

Cymbopogon Martini

PATCHOULI

Note	Base
Botanical Name	Pogostemon Patchouli Pogostemon Cablin
Family	Labiatae
Cultivation	Malaysia, West India, (S.E. Asia), Paraguay
Part of Plant	Leaves
Extracted by	Steam distillation
Yield 1 Gram Oil	Equals 50 grams base material
Constituents	**Alcohol** - Patchoulol **Aldehydes** - Benzoic, Cinnamic **Phenol** - Eugenol **Sesquiterpene** - Cadinene
Principal Constituents	Patchoulol
Adulteration	Cedarwood, Clove Oil and chemicals from Camphor oil, Gurjum balsam oil, Caster oil, etc.
Colour	Dark/orange brown

Aroma	Sweet/balsamic/musky
Blends well with	Bergamot, Geranium, Lavender, Neroli, Rose, Ginger, Frankincense, Lemongrass and Sandalwood
Properties	Fungicide, Insecticide, Sedative, Tonic

MOST COMMON USES

Skin	Acne, Cracked skins
Other	Fungal infections, Dandruff, Obesity, Fluid retention

METHODS OF USE	Local, Massage, Vaporiser, Perfume
CAUTION	Very strong aroma tends to linger which may be disliked. Not to be used on children under the age of 5 years. Reported to cause loss of appetite (caution Anorexia) Reported to be relaxing in low percentage and stimulating in normal percentage.

PATCHOULI

A native shrub of Malaysia although it is now cultivated in China, India, Indonesia and the Seychelles. It grows to about 3ft (1m) in height. This sturdy green, furry leaved shrub bears flowers that are white with the slightest hint of mauve.

The shrub is cropped about twice a year, but it is another of the soil exhausting plants so the soil needs to be well fertilised to maintain the quality.

The Chinese, Japanese and Malaysians have always respected the oil for its powers as an insect repellent. In Victorian times leaves of the plant were placed between the folds of cashmere shawls to protect them from moths. In India the dried leaves or sachets were put into the beds and linen to repel insects and bed bugs.

In view of the fact that some Patchouli is distilled under very primitive conditions without the proper distillation receptacles, the oil may go through some changes through being exposed to certain metals. However there is no evidence to suggest that this process has a detrimental effect on the oil's curative properties. In order to ensure the therapeutic quality of Patchouli it should be purchased only through a professional outlet.

I find the most use for this oil when treating the following conditions:- very oily hair, head lice and as an insect repellent in a house spray.

PATCHOULI

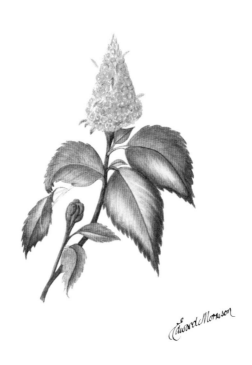

Pogostemon Patchouli

PEPPERMINT

Note	Top
Botanical Name	Mentha Piperita
Family	Labiatae
Cultivation	Europe, Japan, U.S.A.
Part of Plant	Leaves/ Flowering tops
Extracted by	Steam distillation
Yield 1 Gram Oil	Equals 150 grams base material
Constituents	**Alcohol** - Menthol **Ester** - Menthyl acetate, **Ketones** - Carvone, Jasmone, Menthone **Phenol** - Carvacrol **Terpenes** - Limonene, Phellandrene
Principal Constituants	Menthol, Menthone
Adulteration	Unkown
Colour	Pale yellow/ yellow/ green
Aroma	Strong fresh/minty

Blends well with	Lavender, Rosemary, Chamomile, Bergamot, Cypress, Marjoram, Mandarin.
Properties	Antiphlogistic, Carminative, Decongestant, Hepatic, Sudorific

MOST COMMON USES

Digestive	Digestive upsets, Travel sickness, Indigestion
Head	Headaches, Migraine
Other	Sinusitis, Cooling for feverish conditions
METHODS OF USE	Compress, Local massage, Inhalation, Vaporizer
CAUTION	May cause allergic reaction, especially in those prone to sensitivity. Do not use in bath. Do not use on mucouse membrane. Do not use on a client with heart or epeleptic problems or those with a history of convulsions or liver disorder.

NOTE !

There are reports of instant collapse in infants following local application of menthol to their nostrils.

Some schools of thought in the homeopathic profession believe it is best avoided when receiving their treatment as Peppermint can act as an antidote.

PEPPERMINT

A herb that grows to about 3ft (1m). The leaves are serrated and hairy. Pale purple flowers appear from July to September.

Various mint species hybridize naturally and Peppermint is thought to be a hybrid of Mentha Aquatica (Water Mint) and Mentha Spicata (Spearmint).

A native of the Mediterranean it is also cultivated in the U.S.A. and Japan. The first recording of Peppermint cultivation in England was in 1750. Peppermint was known to the ancient Egyptians, Greeks and Romans.

The Hebrews used the oil in their perfumes, which may well have been because of its reputation as an aphrodisiac.

I have found most use for the oil when dealing with digestive problems, abdominal cramps, diarrhoea and constipation.

PEPPERMINT

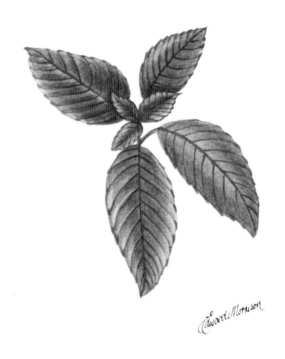

Mentha Piperita

PETITGRAIN

Note	Middle to Top
Botanical Name	Citrus Aurantium
Family	Rutaceae
Cultivation	France, Italy, Spain, North Africa, Paraguay
Part of Plant	Twigs and Leaves
Extracted by	Steam distillation
Yield 1 Gram Oil	Equals 500 grams of base material
Constituents	**Alcohol** - Geraniol, Linalool, Nerol, Terpineol **Esters** - Geranyl acetate, Lynalyl acetate **Terpenes** - Camphene, Limonene
Principal Constituents	Linalyl acetate, Geranyl acetate, Linalool. Over 400 known components in the oil, many of which contribute to the odour
Adulteration	Lemongrass is frequently used to adulterate or substitute for petitgrain, also synthetic citral may be added

Colour	Pale yellowish-orange to brown
Aroma	Floral citrus with woody undertones
Blends well with	Bergamot, Cedarwood, Geranium, Lavender, Neroli, Orange, Palmarosa, Rosemary, Sandlewood, Ylang-Ylang
Properties	Antispasmodic, Antidepressant, Clarifying, Stimulant, Tonic

MOST COMMON USES

Emotional	Anxiety, Depression, Mental fatigue, Stress related conditions
Digestive	Dyspepsia, Flatulence
Skin	Blemishes, Acne
Other	Seems to boost immune system, will aid relaxation and help slow rapid anxious breathing
METHODS OF USE	Bath, Massage, Vaporiser
CAUTION	When adulterated, take lemon oil precautions
NOTE!	Paraguayn Petitgrain is not suitable unless deterpenated first

PETITGRAIN

The name Petitgrain means "little grains" as petitgrain was originally distilled from fruit while still tiny and unripe, rather than the leaves and twigs.

The tree is that of the orange blossom, an evergreen with bright shiny dark green leaves growing to about 30ft (10.5m) high.

The tree displays an abundance of highly scented little white flowers that are picked in May and October to produce Neroli oil. Petitgrain oil is used by both the Pharmaceutical industry and the perfumery profession, the former use it in soft drinks, alcohol and confectionary. The latter used it as a perfume for soaps, detergents and cosmetics.

Petitgrain oil is one of the classic ingredients and smell of eau de cologne.

PETITGRAIN

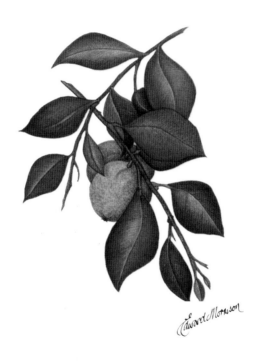

Citrus Aurantium

PINE SCOTCH

Note	Middle
Botanical Name	Pinus Sylvestris
Family	Pinaceae
Cultivation	USA, Europe, Russia Baltic States and Scandinavia
Part of Plant	Needles
Extracted by	Steam distillation
Yield 1 Gram Oil	Equals 50 grams of base material
Constituents	**Alcohol** - Borneol **Esters** - Bornyl acetate, Terpinyl acetate **Sesquiterpene** - Cadinene **Terpenes** - Camphene, Pinene, Chamazulene, Limonene
Principal Constituents	Pinene, Limonene
Adulteration	Mixtures of either natural or synthetic Camphene Pinenes and other chemical components used. May also be mixed with or substituted by inferior oil obtained from wood chippings.
Colour	Colourless/ Pale yellow

Aroma	Strong balsamic, Camphorous.
Blends well with	Eucalyptus, Cedarwood, Tea-Tree, Juniper and Rosemary
Properties	Decongestant, Disinfectant Rubefacient, Stimulant

MOST COMMON USES

Musculoskeletal	Arthritis, Gout, General aches and pains
Nervous	Stress related conditions, Nervous exhaustion, Neuralgia
Genito-Urinary	Cystitis, Urinary infections
Immune System	Colds, Flu
Respiratory	Coughs, Catarrh, Bronchitis, Sinusitis, Asthma
Other	Used to fragrance soaps, detergents, toiletries
METHODS OF USE	Bath, Massage, Inhalation
CAUTION	Avoid sensitive skin types and allergic skin conditions. Ensure oil is fresh as oxidation can cause skin irritation. Do not use in high concentration.

PINE (SCOTCH)

A tall evergreen tree that grows up to 40m tall with a flat top crown. The bark is a reddish brown colour and deeply fissured.
The stiff needles grow in pairs and the brown cones grow pointed.
The oil from the needles of the Scotch Pine is one of the most versatile oils. There are numerous pine trees producing oil, some from the heart of the wood as well as from the needles, and some of the pines are used to produce Turpentine; amongst the uses for Turpentine is that of preserving wood (mainly garden sheds and fences).

Pine has been used to stuff mattresses in order to ward off lice and fleas and it was used by the American Indians to ward off scurvy.
Pine was recognised by the Greeks and Egyptians for its curative powers, particularly for those conditions with connections to the lungs. My grandmother used the twigs to add to the bath for nervous exhaustion and for poor circulation.

I use pine mainly for respiratory disorders and in the vaporiser for sinusitis. I find its refreshing qualities useful in the treatment of rheumatic conditions.

NOTE !
A good household deodoriser.

SCOTCH PINE

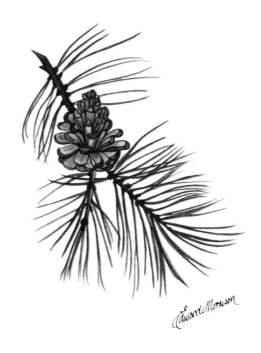

Pinus Sylvestris

ROSE

Note	Middle/Base
Botanical Name	France, Morocco - Rosa Centifolia Bulgaria - Rosa Damascena (Otto)
Family	Rosaceae
Cultivation	Bulgaria, Morocco, France
Part of Plant	Flowers
Extracted by	Enfleurage / Steam distillation
Yield 1 Gram Oil	Equals approximately 4000 grams base material
Constituents	**Acid** - Geranic **Alcohol** - Citronellol, Geraniol, Farnesol, Nerol **Phenol** - Eugenol **Terpene** - Myrcene
Principal Constituents	Citronellol, Geraniol 70% of the Rose aroma is given to the oil by Damascenone found in the oil at only 0.14%
Adulteration	Common due to cost of true Rose Oil and even Rose Absolute may be adulterated. Sophisticated methods of adulteration make detection difficult.

Colour	Pale/yellow, orange/ brown, orange/green
Aroma	Rich floral
Blends well with	Many oils especially Bergamot, Clary-Sage, Geranium, Jasmine, Patchouli, Sandalwood, Lavender, Chamomile.
Properties	Antidepressant, Aphrodisiac, Feminine, Sedative

MOST COMMON USES

Regulating female cycle, Post-natal depression, Grief, Skin care (all types). Rose oil is often considered to be the feminine oil suitable for all female related problems. Under normal circumstances this oil should be used in one of the following dilutions :

1 % =1 drop - 5ml Carrier
½% =1 drop - 10ml Carrier
¼% =1 drop - 20ml Carrier

METHODS OF USE

Bath, Compress, Massage, Skin treatment products, Vapouriser, Perfume

CAUTION

A strong aroma usually dictates a lower percentage use in Aromatherapy massage

ROSE

The Rose hardly needs description. It is cultivated throughout the world (originally native to the Orient) growing on its thorny shrubs. The Damask Rose (Rosa Damascena) for example, has leaves which are glossy on top and hairy underneath. It has small pink, white or red flowers arranged in coryubs (pendicles are different lengths so all flowers are the same level at the top, the outer flowers opening first).

The Rose has been prized throughout history for the colour and shape of the bloom but above all for the nature of its scent. The Ancient Egyptians used roses in religious ceremonies. Roses have been found in the tombs next to the Mummies.

The art of distilling Rose oil originated in Persia. The Persian warriors adorned their shields with red roses (the symbol of Persia at the time). The Romans hung roses from the ceilings during banquets and wore them to protect themselves from drunkenness (they drank Rosewater for the same purpose).

During the 17th century Bulgaria began the commercial production of Rose oil. The Bulgarians were for some considerable time the world's main producers, though Morocco and Turkey now produce vast quantities.

Rose Otto oil is the more expensive but also the more effective in therapy. The reason for the expense is twofold; first the low yield of essential oil from roses (100 times less than the average yield from other plants), secondly the Rose blooms for just 30 days and needs to be hand picked in the early morning during July and August. Sunshine evaporates the oil from the flower so the oil content drops. When the roses have been collected the flowers must be processed within 24 hours.

ROSE

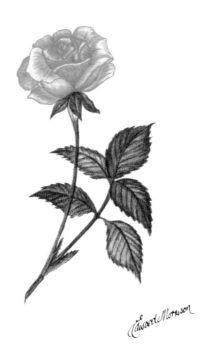

Rosa Centifolia

ROSEMARY

Note	Middle
Botanical Name	Rosmarinus Officinalis
Family	Labiatae
Cultivation	France, Spain, Tunisia
Part of Plant	Flowering tops and leaves
Extracted by	Steam distillation
Yield 1 Gram Oil	Equals 70 grams base material
Constituents	**Alcohol** - Borneol **Aldehyde** - Cuminic **Ester** - Bornyl acetate **Ketones** - Camphor **Oxide** - Cineole **Terpenes** - Camphene, Pinene. **Sesquiterpene** - Caryophyllene
Principal Constituents	Cineole
Adulteration	Mixed with or substituted with Camphor, Cypress, Eucalyptus. Spanish Sage and synthetic fractions may also be used.
Colour	Pale yellow
Aroma	Fresh/camphorous

Blends well with	Citrus oils, Frankincense, Lavender, Peppermint, Cedarwood, Geranium and Ginger
Properties	Analgesic, Antispasmodic, Cephalic, Rubefacient, Stimulant

MOST COMMON USES

Digestive	Constipation/Liver/Gall bladder
Head	Poor memory Hair loss
Musculoskeletal	Aches and pains, Arthritis, Rheumatism
Respiratory	Asthma, Chronic bronchitis
METHODS OF USE	Bath, Compress, Massage, Vaporizer, Inhalation (from hankie)
CAUTION	Not to be used in cases of high blood pressure or on epileptics.

ROSEMARY

An evergreen shrub which grows to about 3ft (1m) high. It is native to the Mediterranean but is cultivated widely elsewhere.

The plant has a pleasant camphor-like smell and flowers from May to August. The stem is woody and branched, the leaves linear, about 1.5cm to 2.5cm long with resolute margins (bent back at the edges). The leaf is green on top with a whitish underneath. Flower colour is a bluish-lilac.

My main use for this oil is for mental fatigue and local areas of aches and pains.

ROSEMARY

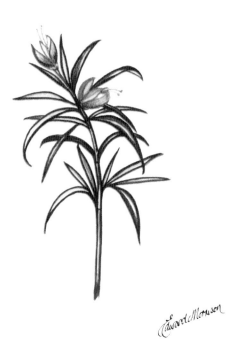

Rosmarinus Officinalis

SANDALWOOD

Note	Base
Botanical Name	Santalum Album
Family	Santalaceae
Cultivation	East India
Part of Plant	Heart wood
Extracted by	Steam distillation
Yield 1 Gram Oil	Equals 25 grams base material
Constituents	**Alcohol** - Santalol **Aldehyde** - Furfurul **Sesquiterpene** - Santalene
Principal Constituents	Santalol, Santelene
Adulteration	Amyris Oil, Cedarwood oil, Castor oil and similar often added. Odourless solvents may also be used, e.g. Liquid paraffin, Glyceryl acetate, Benzyl alcohol. Synthetic substitutes Sandela and Sandalore may be used due to cheapness.
Colour	Pale/dark yellow
Aroma	Rich woody

Blends well with	Black Pepper, Cypress, Neroli, Bergamot, Lemon, Frankincense, Ylang-Ylang, Lavender and many others.
Properties	Antidepressant, Antiphlogistic, Carminative, Emollient

MOST COMMON USES

Emotional	Nervous tension, Depression, Insomnia
Digestive	Diarrhoea, Nausea, Colic
Skin Care	All types
Respiratory	Catarrh, Bronchitis
Other	Cystitis
METHODS OF USE	Bath, Compress, Massage, Vaporizer, Perfume
CAUTION	Specific not known but as with all oils exercise caution especially as there may be adulteration.

SANDALWOOD

Sandalwood is a small evergreen tree which takes approximately fifty years to reach full maturity, at which point it will have reached a height of 50ft (15m). The young grey/white trunk varies in colour as the tree matures, finally becoming yellow/orange colour. The many slender branches have oval, leathery leaves and small, pinky purple flowers.

This lovely tree starts life as a semi-parasite germinating from the black seeds of the mother tree. Roots attach themselves to nearby trees or bushes and for the next seven years the young tree depends on its host for nourishment, (eventually causing it to die); at which stage the new tree can survive and grow on its own. Sandalwood must be at least 30 years of age before it can be cut down to produce oil. The oil is obtained mainly from the heart wood though some is also produced from the roots. A fully grown tree can yield up to 200kg (440lbs) of oil.

Sandalwood was used by the Egyptians both in medicine and embalming. The Indians used it for skin infections, abscesses, etc. In 1868 Dr. Henderson (a Glaswegian doctor), mentioned its benefits for Blennoragia (discharge of mucus). This research was later confirmed by no less than three french doctors. During this period Sandalwood was used mainly for general urinary problems. In China it was used for stomach ache.

Although the tree has had about 4000 years of use many therapists are now concerned about the increased demand for the oil in the cosmetic and perfumery business; which in turn is causing vast areas to be robbed of trees.

Sandalwood will always be a favourite oil but my love of nature and my alarm at present day destruction limits my use of this oil to rare occasions.

SANDALWOOD

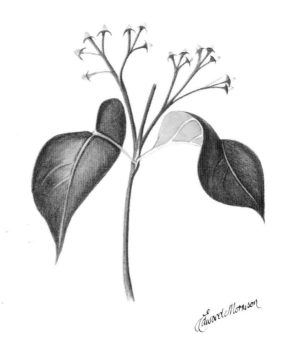

Santalum Album

TANGERINE

Note	Top/Middle
Botanical Name	Citrus Reticulata
Family	Rutaceae
Cultivated	China, USA, Sicily
Part of Plant	Peel
Extracted by	Expression
Yield 1 Gram Oil	Equals 150 grams of base material
Constituents	**Alcohols** - Citronellol, Linalool **Aldehyde** - Citral **Sesquiterpene** - Cadinene **Terpene** - Limonene
Principal Constituents	Limonene
Adulteration	Other citrus oils especially citrus oil terpenes or addition of synthetic Limonene. Antioxidants may be added to increase shelf life
Colour	Golden
Aroma	Tangy/ slightly sweet

Blends well with	All oils
Properties	Antispasmodic, Cholagogue,Cytophylactic, Digestive, Sedative, Tonic
MOST COMMON USES	Depression, Convalescence, Digestion, PMT, All skin types, Children
Other	Blending- Adding 1% to the total floral mix makes a pleasing,less heavy, heady smell (flower oils used alone can be overpowering)
METHODS OF USE	Bath, Compress, Massage, Vapouriser
CAUTION	It may be phototoxic so exercise care and avoid sun/sunbed for 12 hours before and after use.

TANGERINE

The Tangerine is very similar to the Mandarin. A native of China, it was brought to America in the mid 19th century.

The fruit, which is smaller than an orange, is very similar to the Mandarin though more orange in colour with no pips.

Considered by some therapists to be the most suitable oil for use in pregnancy.

I use the oil as I would Mandarin:

Children
People convalescing
New mothers
All skin types
Blending with other oils, especially the heavy florals to make less heavy, heady oils.

I do not use this oil if the skin shows signs of Melanoma, Pre-Melanoma, large dark moles or any skin Cancers.

TANGERINE

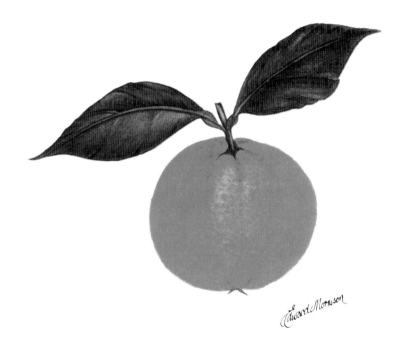

Citrus Reticulata

THYME

Note	Top/Middle
Botanical Name	Thymus Vulgaris
Family	Labiatae
Cultivation	Mediterranean
Part of Plant	Flowering tops
Extracted by	Steam distillation
Yield 1 Gram Oil	Equals 100 grams base material
Constituents	**Alcohols** - Borneol, Linalool **Phenols** - Thymol, Carvacrol **Terpenes** - Terpinene Cymene **Sesquiterpene** - Caryophyllene
Principal Constituents	Thymol approximately 60% in white and 50% in red. Thyme may have a high Carvacrol content.
Adulteration	Common - Organum and various thyme oils. Fractions Eucalyptus and Rosemary. There is a wide variety of Thyme oil available.

Colour	Red or white. Red more commonly used in Aromatherapy.
Aroma	Sweetish / strong herbal.
Blends well with	Bergamot, Chamomile, Cedarwood, Juniper, Melissa, Rosemary and Tea-Tree.
Properties	Antirheumatic, Antiseptic, Antispasmodic, Aphrodisiac, Bactericide, Bechic, Carminative, Cicatrisant, Diuretic, Emmenagogue, Expectorant, Insecticide, Stimulant, Tonic, Vermifuge

MOST COMMON USES

Emotional	Concentration, Memory, Depression, Exhaustion
Respiratory	Bronchitis, Tonsillitis
Circulatory	Low blood pressure
Other	Arthritic swelling, Rheumatism, Gout

METHODS OF USE	Local Massage, Vaporiser
CAUTION	Due to adulteration caution is absolutely necessary.

THYME

There are 3,000 species of Thyme; it is believed all or most originated from wild Thyme, a perennial evergreen shrub which grows to a height of 11-18 inches (45cm). The Thyme shrub has small oval leaves, a woody root and branched upright stems. The flowers vary in colour from white or pale pink through to purple and deep red. Thyme also varies in scent from caraway or orange to mint.

Thyme has a long history and myth has it that the herb was born from the tears of Helen of Troy. Egyptians used it in the embalming process and in the days of epidemics judges carried sprigs into the courtroom to ward off infection.

Thyme is a powerful oil and should therefore be used with caution.

My main use for this oil is in the treatment of Rheumatism, Arthritis and infections.

THYME

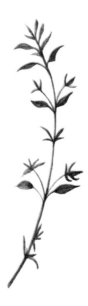

Thymus Vulgaris

TEA-TREE

Note	Top
Botanical Name	Melaleuca Alternifolia
Family	Myrtaceae
Cultivation	Australia
Part of Plant	Leaves
Extracted by	Steam distillation
Yield 1 Gram Oil	Equals 90 grams base material
Constituents	**Alcohol** - Terpinenol **Keytone** - Cineole **Terpenes** - Cymene, Pinene, Terpinene
Principal Constituents	Cineole, Terpinene approximately 30%
Adulteration	Using oil from various species
Colour	Yellow
Aroma	Camphorous/balsamic
Blends well with	Few oils. Best with Lavender, Lemon, Cypress, Rosemary, Mandarin and Chamomile
Properties	Antifungal, Antiviral, Insecticide

MOST COMMON USES

Digestive	Gastroenteritis
Head	Mouth wash, Cold sores, Dandruff
Respiratory	Sinusitis, Bronchitis
Skin	Candida, Insect bites, Acne, Verruca, Athlete's foot, Warts, Chicken pox, Shingles, Boils, Rashes
Other	Insect repellent and household spray when flu is about

METHODS OF USE	Bath, Compress, Massage, Vaporizer, Alcohol base

CAUTION	Cineole is a known skin sensitiser. Australian Standards Commission ensure maximum Cineole is 15% in Tea-Tree oil. In reality it is more usual to be around 5% in Melaleuca Alternifolia.

NOTE !

Some therapists are reporting skin sensitivity. This may be due to oil quality or overuse especially on damaged skin.

TEA-TREE

A small tree (Melaleuca Altrenifolia) native to Australia which grows to about 20ft (6-7m). It is similar in appearance to the Cypress with needle-like leaves and creamy-yellowish flowers.

The Tea-Tree has remarkable powers of recuperation and if it is chopped down to the stump it will grow again very quickly.

The oil is obtained from the leaves and is one of the more valuable oils for treating infections and a variety of skin conditions.

The oil has a history with the Aboriginal people of Australia and was one of the bush remedies used by early settlers. Tea-Tree was a remedy in the first aid kits of the Australian army and navy during the Second World War. After the war however, progression in the use of the oil slowed down and it was not until the early 70's that Tea-Tree returned to the forefront of essential oil awareness. It is now a most valued oil in Aromatherapy, although for some it may be a skin irritant.

For me Tea-Tree is a very necessary oil being antibacterial, antiviral and antifungal. I use Tea-Tree for the following conditions: Athlete's foot, thrush (candida), warts/verrucae, herpes simplex (cold sores), shingles, chickenpox, acne and patients with AIDS related skin conditions.

TEA-TREE

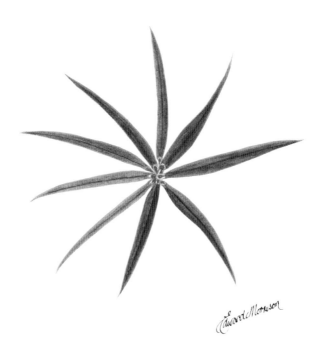

Melaleuca Alternifolia

VIOLET

Note	Middle
Botanical Name	Viola Odorata
Family	Violaceae
Cultivation	France, Italy, Egypt, China
Part of Plant	Flowers / Leaves
Extracted by	Enfleurage
Yield 1 gram	Equals 700 grams of base material
Constituents	**Acid** - Salicylic **Alcohol** - Benzyl **Ketone** - Parmone **Phenol** - Eugenol
Principal Constituants	Benzyl alcohol, Salicylic acid.
Adulteration	Mix of leaf and flower oil. May have Ylang-Ylang added and or Synthetic components.
Colour	Flower - Yellowish/green Leaf - Dark green
Aroma	Flower - Sweet rich floral Leaf - Strong green-leaf

Blends well with	Frankincense, Sandalwood, Orange, Grapefruit, Lemon, Jasmine and Rose
Properties	Analgesic, (mild) Anti-inflamatory, Antiseptic, Diuretic, Laxative, Circulation (stimulant), Expectorant

MOST COMMON USES

Skin	Acne, Refines pores
Respiratory	Mouth/Throat infections, Bronchitis
Circulation	Thread veins
Nervous	Nervous exhaution, Insomnia, Headaches
Urinary	Diuretic
Digestive	Sluggish, Constipation

METHODS OF USE	Bath, Compress, Massage, Perfume, Vapouriser
CAUTION	Possible sensitisation in some susceptible people

NOTE !
Violet has a very pleasing floral smell and as such is used in some of the most expensive perfumes.

VIOLET

The violet is a small popular perennial garden plant with dark green heart shaped leaves and blue to violet fragrant flowers.

The Anglo Saxons thought it a good remedy against evil spirits. The ancient Greeks used it as a symbol for fertility. In the 19th century hot violet leaves were used to ease the pain of tumours. In the late 19th century sweets were made to ease chest problems. My grandmother and mother made violet skin complexion milk with an infusion of flowers in goat's milk.

Two types of Violet are used in the perfumery industry; Parma preferred for its delicate scent and the Victoriana, the hardier of the two species. Violet perfume was the most favoured perfume of Marie Antoinette.

I still occasionally use my grandmother's recipe for my own skin. In the clinic I find violet most useful for relaxation, general sluggish systems and congested skins. The perfume, when blended with citrus or woods, makes a very pleasing aroma for either male or female clients.

VIOLET

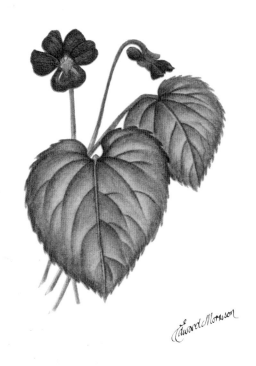

Viola Odorata

YLANG-YLANG

Note	Middle/Base
Botanical Name	Cananga Odorata
Family	Anonaceae
Cultivation	Madagascar, Java, Sumatra and Comoro Islands
Part of Plant	Flowers
Extracted by	Steam distillation
Yield 1 Gram Oil	Equals 100 grams base material
Constituents	**Acid** - Benzoic **Alcohols** - Farnesol, Geraniol, Linalool **Ester** - Benzyl acetate **Phenols** - Eugenol, Safrol **Sesquiterpene** - Cadinene **Terpene** - Pinene
Principal Constituents	Geraniol, Linalool
Adulteration	Cananga Oil may be added or substituted. Synthetic components may also be added.
Colour	Pale yellow
Aroma	Spicy/floral

Blends well with	Sandalwood, Jasmine, Bergamot, Lemon Frankincense and many more.
Properties	Antidepressant, Hypotensive

MOST COMMON USES

Emotional	Depression, Insomnia, Frigidity, Tension, Anxiety, Stress
Other	Rapid heart beat, Rapid breathing, High blood pressure , Epilepsy

METHODS OF USE	Bath, Massage, Vaporizer, Perfume
CAUTION	May be sensitising on skins prone to Dermatitis/Eczema type conditions. Some reports of headaches after use which may possibly be due to the powerful aroma of the oil. Do not use in cases of low blood pressure.

NOTE !   Unless sure of the purity use in low dilutions. Cananga Oil is used to adulterate some Ylang-Ylang and is a known skin irritant.

YLANG-YLANG

A native of the tropics, especially Indonesia, Madagascar and the Philippines, the Ylang-Ylang tree grows to 66ft (20m).

The branches bend slightly downwards showing large sweet scented yellowish-white flowers and huge, oval, shiny leaves. The wild Ylang-Ylang blossom has very little aroma.

The best quality oil comes from the Philippines but unfortunately oils from this area seem to be on the decline and an inferior quality oil from a slightly different tree which grows abundantly in Java is being sold as Ylang-Ylang, or as an alternative for Ylang-Ylang and is known only as Cananga.

Ylang-Ylang was first mentioned in the 17th century by an english botanist John Ray. It was used in a hair oil known as Macassar in Victorian times. One thing the famous hair oil did was to stain chair and sofa backs so much that washable covers, called Antimacassars were devised for the furniture.

Like Jasmine, Rose and Sandalwood, Ylang-Ylang is considered to be an aphrodisiac.

In the treatment of my clients I have found Ylang-Ylang most useful for the following conditions : depression; PMS; menopausal symptoms; anxiety; shock; frigidity; anger; high blood pressure, rapid heartbeat and epilepsy.

YLANG YLANG

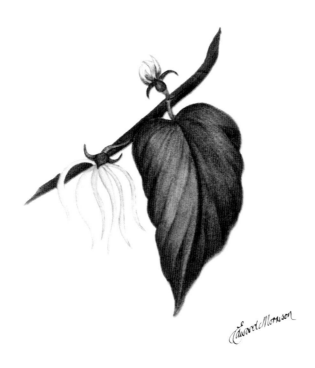

Cananga Odorata

DIRECTORY OF DEFINITIONS AND INDEX OF PROPERTIES

Analgesic :   Reduces pain

Anaphrodisiac :   Decreases sexual response

Antiallergenic :   Reduces allergic sensitivity

Anticonvulsive: Relieves convulsions

Antidepressant: Helps to lift the mood

Antiemetic: Helps to prevent vomiting

Antirheumatic: Helps to relieve the symptoms of rheumatism

Anti-Inflammatory: Reduces inflammation

Antiphlogistic: Counteracts inflammation

Antipruritic:	Eliminates itching
Antineuralgic:	Helps relieve neuralgic symptoms
Antiscorbutic:	Counteracts the effects of scurvy
Antiseptic:	Prevents or combats bacterial infection
Antispasmodic:	Relieves smooth-muscle spasm
Antitoxic:	Counteracts poisoning
Antiviral:	Inhibits growth/activity of viruses
Aphrodisiac:	Increases sexual response
Astringent:	Tightens tissues
Bactericide:	Kills bacteria
Balsamic:	Qualities of a restorative balm (healing)

Bechic: Eases coughing

Carminative: Prevents/relieves flatulence

Cephalic: Clears the mind
Stimulates mental activity

Cholagogue: Stimulates the flow of bile

Cicatrisant: Promotes formation of scar tissue

Cordial: Generally invigorating and
stimulating

Cytophylactic: Cell regenerator

Decongestant: Relieves congestion

Deodorant: Reduces odour

Detoxicant: Helps cleanse body of impurities

Digestive: Aids digestion of food

Depurative:	Assists in effecting purification
Diuretic:	Increases production of urine
Emmenagogue:	Encourages menstruation
Emollient:	Skin or mucous membrane softener
Expectorant:	Helps expulsion of phlegm
Febrifuge:	Reduces fever
Fungicide:	Kills or inhibits growth of yeast, moulds, etc:
Galactagogue:	Increases the flow of milk
Haemostatic:	Checks bleeding
Hepatic:	Strengthens liver
Hypertensive:	Raises blood pressure

Hypnotic:	Induces sleep
Hypotensive:	Lowers blood pressure
Immunostimulant:	Strengthens the body's defence system to infection
Insecticide:	Repels insects
Laxative:	Promotes bowel evacuation
Nervine:	Strengthens the nervous system
Parturient:	Promotes and eases labour
Rubefacient:	Produces warmth and redness to the skin
Sedative:	Calming action on the nervous system
Splenetic:	Tonic for the spleen
Stomachic:	Stomach stimulant

Stimulant: Increases activity of the body or organ

Sudorific: Promotes sweating

Tonic: Strengthens the body or organ

Uterine: Tonic action on the womb

Vasoconstrictor: Helps small blood vessels contract

Vasodilator: Helps small blood vessels expand

Vulnerary: Helps wounds to heal

SOME PROPERTIES OF ESSENTIAL OILS

Basil
Cephalic
Tonic
Emmenagogue
Sudorific

Benzoin
Carminative
Expectorant
Deodorant
Sedative
Diuretic
Vulnerary

Bergamot
Analgesic
Antiseptic
Digestive
Sedative
Antidepressant
Bactericide
Expectorant
Vulnerary
Anti-Inflammatory
Deodorant
Febrifuge

Black Pepper
Analgesic
Antitoxic
Detoxicant
Febrifuge
Stimulant
Antiseptic
Aphrodisiac
Digestive
Laxative
Stomachic
Antispasmodic
Carminative
Diuretic
Rubefacient
Tonic

Cajuput
Analgesic
Antispasmodic
Cicatrisant
Febrifuge
Sudorific
Antineuralgic
Bactericide
Decongestant
Insecticide
Antirheumatic
Balsamic
Expectorant
Stimulant

Calendula
Anti-inflammatory
Fungicide

Chamomile
Analgesic
Antidepressant
Antiphlogistic
Diuretic
Febrifuge
Nervine
Sudorific
Vulnerary

Antiallergenic
Antiemetic
Antipruritic
Emmenagogue
Hepatic
Sedative
Tonic

Anticonvulsive
Anti-inflammatory
Cholagogue
Emollient
Hypnotic
Splenic
Vasoconstrictor

Cedarwood
Astringent
Expectorant
Tonic

Diuretic
Insecticide

Emollient
Sedative

Cinnamon
Antiseptic
Astringent
Haemostatic
Stomachic

Antispasmodic
Carminative
Insecticide
Vermifuge

Aphrodisiac
Emmenagogue
Stimulant

Clary Sage
Anticonvulsive
Antispasmodic
Carminative
Emmenagogue
Parturient
Uterine

Antidepressant
Aphrodisiac
Deodorant
Hypotensive
Sedative

Antiphlogistic
Balsamic
Digestive
Nervine
Tonic

Cypress
Antirheumatic
Cicatrisant
Febrifuge
Insecticide
Vasoconstrictor

Antispasmodic
Deodorant
Haemostatic
Sedative

Astringent
Diuretic
Hepatic
Tonic

Eucalyptus

Analgesic	Antiphlogistic	Antirheumatic
Antiseptic	Antispasmodic	Antiviral
Bactericide	Cicatrisant	Decongestant
Deodorant	Diuretic	Expectorant
Febrifuge	Insecticide	Rubefacient
Stimulant	Vulnerary	

Frankincense

Astringent	Digestive	Diuretic
Sedative	Tonic	

Fennel Sweet

Antiphlogistic	Antispasmodic	Detoxicant
Diuretic	Emmenagogue	Expectorant

Geranium

Analgesic	Antidepressant	Astringent
Cicatrisant	Cytophylactic	Deodorant
Diuretic	Haemostatic	Insecticide
Stimulant	Tonic	Vasoconstrictor
Vulnerary		

Ginger

Analgesic	Antidepressant	Antiemetic
Antiscorbutic	Antiseptic	Aphrodisiac
Carminative	Expectorant	Febrifuge
Laxative	Rubefacient	Stimulant
Stomachic	Sudorific	Tonic

Grapefruit

Antidepressant	Digestive	Stimulant
Tonic		

Jasmine

Antidepressant	Antirheumatic	Antispasmodic
Aphrodisiac	Emollient	Parturient
Sedative	Uterine	

Juniper

Antiseptic	Antispasmodic	Antirheumatic
Astringent	Bactericide	Carminative
Cicatrisant	Detoxicant	Diuretic
Emmenagogue	Insecticide	Nervine
Parturient	Rubefacient	Sedative
Stimulant	Sudorific	Tonic
Vulnerary		

Lavender

Analgesic	Anticonvulsive	Antidepressant
Anti-Inflammatory	Antiphlogistic	Antirheumatic
Antiseptic	Antispasmodic	Antiviral
Bactericide	Bechic	Carminative
Cholagogue	Cicatrisant	Cordial
Cytophylactic	Decongestant	Deodorant
Detoxicant	Diuretic	Emmenagogue
Fungicide	Hypnotic	Hypotensive
Immuno-Stimulant	Nervine	Sedative
Splenic	Sudorific	Tonic
Vulnerary		

Lemon

Antineuralgic	Antipruritic	Antirheumatic
Antiscorbutic	Antiseptic	Astringent
Bactericide	Carminative	Cicatrisant
Diuretic	Emollient	Febrifuge
Haemostatic	Hepatic	Insecticide
Laxative	Tonic	

Lemongrass

Antidepressant	Antiseptic	Bactericide
Carminative	Deodorant	Diuretic
Fungicide	Insecticide	Stimulant
Tonic		

Lime

Antiscorbutic	Antiseptic	Antiviral
Astringent	Bactericide	Disinfectant
Febrifuge	Haemostatic	Insecticide
Restorative	Tonic	

Mandarin

Antispasmodic	Cholagogue	Cytophylactic
Digestive	Emollient	Sedative
Tonic		

Marjoram

Analgesic	Anaphrodisiac	Antiseptic
Antispasmodic	Carminative	Cephalic
Cordial	Digestive	Emmenagogue
Expectorant	Hypotensive	Hypnotic
Laxative	Nervine	Sedative
Tonic	Vasodilator	Vulnerary

Melissa

Antiallergenic	Antidepressant	Antispasmodic
Carminative	Cordial	Digestive
Febrifuge	Hypotensive	Nervine
Sedative	Tonic	Uterine

Myrrh

Anti-Inflammatory	Astringent	Emmenagogue
Expectorant	Fungicide	Sedative
Tonic	Uterine tonic	Vulnerary

Neroli

Antidepressant
Bactericide
Cytophylactic
Emollient
Tonic

Antispasmodic
Carminative
Deodorant
Hypnotic

Aphrodisiac
Cordial
Digestive
Sedative

Niouli

Analgesic
Balsamic
Decongestant
Stimulant

Antirheumatic
Bactericide
Febrifuge
Vulnerary

Antiseptic
Cicatrisant
Insecticide

Patchouli

Antidepressant
Aphrodisiac
Cytophylactic
Febrifuge
Sedative

Antiphlogistic
Astringent
Deodorant
Fungicide
Tonic

Antiseptic
Cicatrisant
Diuretic
Insecticide

Peppermint

Analgesic
Astringent
Cordial
Expectorant
Nervine
Vasoconstrictor

Antiphlogistic
Cephalic
Decongestant
Febrifuge
Stimulant

Antispasmodic
Cholagogue
Emmenagogue
Hepatic
Sudorific

Petitgrain

Antidepressant
Sedative

Antispasmodic

Deodorant

Pine

Antiphlogistic	Antiseptic	Balsamic
Decongestant	Deodorant	Disinfectant
Diuretic	Expectorant	Restorative
Rubefacient	Stimulant	Sudorific
Tonic		

Rose

Antidepressant	Antiphlogistic	Antispasmodic
Aphrodisiac	Astringent	Bactericide
Cholagogue	Depurative	Diuretic
Emmenagogue	Haemostatic	Hepatic
Laxative	Sedative	Splenic
Tonic	Uterine tonic	Vasoconstrictor

Rosemary

Analgesic	Antidepressant	Antirheumatic
Antiseptic	Antispasmodic	Astringent
Bactericide	Cephalic	Cholagogue
Cicatrisant	Cordial	Digestive
Diuretic	Emmenagogue	Hepatic
Hypertensive	Nervine	Rubefacient
Stimulant	Sudorific	Tonic
Vulnerary		

Sandalwood

Antidepressant	Antiphlogistic	Antiseptic
Antispasmodic	Aphrodisiac	Astringent
Bechic	Diuretic	Emollient
Expectorant	Sedative	Tonic

Tangerine

Antispasmodic	Cholagogue	Cytophlactic
Sedative	Tonic	

Tea-Tree

Antiseptic	Antiviral	Bactericide
Balsamic	Cicatrisant	Cordial
Cytophylactic	Expectorant	Febrifuge
Fungicide	Immuno-Stimulant	Insecticide
Stimulant	Sudorific	Tonic
Vulnerary		

Thyme

Antirheumatic	Antispasmodic	Aphrodisiac
Bactericide	Bechic	Cicatrisant
Diuretic	Emmenagogue	Expectorant
Hypertensive	Insecticide	Stimulant
Tonic		

Violet

Antidepressant	Antiseptic	Aphrodisiac
Bechic	Diuretic	Expectorant
Laxative	Sedative	

Ylang-Ylang

Antidepressant	Antiseptic	Aphrodisiac
Hypnotic	Hypotensive	Sedative

CLIENT CARE

The Aromatherapist needs to be professional, caring, understanding and sympathetic. They must have the wisdom to understand when medical advice should be sought and never make claims for cures or give false hope. Neither can any guarantees be given as each blend and client is different. The professional therapist will also know that there are some oils that would never be used under any circumstances. Training will teach, all things having been considered, the most suitable oil for a particular client.

The atmosphere where the client is treated needs to be warm and relaxing with a subdued light and a subtle aroma of essential oils; the surroundings and the attitude of the therapist will have an immediate effect on the client.

When the client arrives the therapist will take his or her coat or show them where to put it. It is important for the client to be taken care of as soon as they arrive and that the therapist concentrates on the needs of that client. In order to do this the client has to be made to feel comfortable, be offered a seat and have the general treatment explained before the therapist starts off on a lengthy questionnaire on medical history and lifestyle.

Reasons for the consultation/questionnaire should be explained to the client (e.g. a holistic approach); also the fact that blending is to suit individual needs and lifestyle. It should be established that there are no contra-indications (reasons why treatment cannot be performed). The client should then be asked if they would like to use the toilet. On returning to the treatment room the client is asked to undress (preferably behind a screen) and given a bath sheet to wrap in. When the client is ready, the therapist guides them to the couch and indicates whether they should lay face down on the couch or otherwise depending on treatment.

Some Aromatherapists ask the clients to undress completely, although naturally the client's wishes should be considered. It would not be possible to give a full body massage when the client is wearing an all-in-one. Personally I feel it would be easier to carry out the treatment on the back and shoulders on a female client if she removes her bra. Where the client feels shy or embarrassed a good therapist will work by undoing the fastening and moving the straps off the shoulders, (when the client is lying prone on couch) prior to commencing massage of the back. There is still a danger of either the client or the therapist getting oil on the bra, (something which the therapist should explain to the client). If a pair of knickers or underpants are worn by the client they can be protected with a paper towel. Whatever the circumstance the client should always be given a modesty towel).

The client should be given a glass of water after treatment as the first step in the cleansing process from within. The water also helps to make the client feel fresh and hydrated which will give an uplifted feeling.

WINDOWS AND DOORS

CLOSING
It is advisable to close the windows and doors while giving a treatment because the room should be comfortable and warm to ensure client relaxation during the treatment. If the windows and doors are left open some of the odiferous molecules from the oils will escape and therefore the impact of the oils on the olfactory nerves in the nose of the client will be lessened.

OPENING
The windows and doors should be open between treatments in order to keep the room fresh and eliminate the build up of odours.

A Typical Consultation Card

THERAPIST'S NAME
Name   Name of Doctor
Address   Address
Telephone Number   Tel. Nunber
Date of Birth
Weight
Height
Occupation
Referred by
Reason for visit
Tel. No. Next of Kin (relationship)

Known Medical History
Medication
Previous Illnesses
Family Illnesses
Previous Operations
Accidents/Injuries
Back Problems
Allergies Self/Family
Menstrual Problems (F)
SkinType
State of Health General

Lifestyle
No.of Children
Ages of Children
Marital status
Smoking (amount)
Drinking (amount)
Balanced Diet
Eating Habits
RegularExercise
Work Routine
Sleep Pattern
Stress Prone-effects of
Depression Prone-effects of

Other
Physical difficulties
Eyesight
Hearing
Posture
Any other condition, disorder or disease you would like to discuss.

Are you currently receiving any other form of therapy?
Last visit to GP   Reason
Last visit to Hospital   Reason

CLIENT'S SIGNATURE   **THERAPIST'S SIGNATURE**
                                        Date

REACTIONS TO OILS

Some abnormal reactions that can occur during or immediately after treatment:
1. Nausea
2. Headaches
3. Anxiety
4. Unable to sleep
5. Itching (extreme)
6. Swelling (extreme)
7. Fainting (extreme)
Occasionally some of the above reactions may be due to the therapist choosing the incorrect oil rather than the client's abnormal reaction.

Abnormal reactions can occur in anyone, especially the following groups:
1. Elderly
2. Children
3. Breast feeding mothers
4. Allergy sufferers
6. Asthmatics
7. Epileptics
8. Pregnancy
Pregnancy needs special care. I personally do not use essential oils in pregnancy other than citrus oils. If you are considering doing so then see a professional for advice (students discuss with tutor).
See page 341

For the above more susceptible groups use oils in a more diluted form, increasing to the desired quantity only when you are convinced there is no risk.

HINTS FOR THE THERAPIST

1. Give each client a full consultation on their first visit using a pre-prepared typed professional record sheet (NOT A SMALL CARD). Allow about half an hour for this consultation, check medical history and lifestyle. On each return visit read the consultation sheet checking if any changes have occurred. On the first visit the reason for the consultation/ questionnaire should be explained and the client should be reassured that the information given to the therapist is confidential. The therapist should ask the questions and do the writing, after which the client should read and sign the consultation sheet with help from the therapist if necessary.

2. Explain the treatment expectations and limitations as well as what you intend to do on this visit, e.g. full body massage, treat back only, etc.

3. Ask client if he/she would like to use the toilet and show them where it is. Do not create stress by sending them on a search and find mission.

4. Explain exactly which clothing needs to be removed and which can stay on. Offer to help the elderly or less able. Ask client to remove jewellery and place it in their shoe or his/her bag. For security reasons the client should do this themselves.

5. Allow client to undress in private (if there is only one room then keep busy preparing the oils and buy a screen as a priority).

6. Explain to the client how you would like him/her to lie down on the couch, e.g. "on the tummy, head this end." Help the client by guiding with your hand.

7. Unless weather is very mild use warm towels to cover the client and keep the room at a comfortable temperature.

8. Check that the chosen oils are not contra indicated to any condition/ disorder on your consultation sheet/questionnaire.
Use smelling strips, blotting paper or a cotton bud to let the client smell the aroma of your mix and don't drop or drip on the clothes.

9. Wash hands before and after treatment making client aware that you are doing so.

10. Give the treatment. Keep to allotted time. The client may be busy; perhaps have a car in a parking bay or may need to get a meal ready. He/she may like your treatments but will not return to you if you keep them over time.

11. Do not discuss politics, religion or sex. They tend to be emotive subjects. Do not gossip, ask only relevant questions in the consultation. Do not be nosey. Allow the client to sleep or talk during treatment, whichever seems best for them. Do not discuss your other clients.

12. Remember the client is paying for your professional knowledge not to listen to your problems. Keep your own problems for your friends or go and see a professional.

13. When treatment is complete help the client off the couch, wrap in a towel and sit them on a nearby chair.

14. Go and wash your hands. On your return bring two glasses of water; one for you and one for the client. Give an explanation to the client why he/she should drink water.

15. Allow the client to dress in private or help if necessary. The therapist could use any free time now to complete record cards or prepare homecare preparations if required.

16. Give client a price list and any relevant publicity material.

17. Make next appointment. Try to keep to the same day and time, the client is less likely to forget. It is acceptable to remind the client to make the diary entry.

18. Throughout the treatment the client should be made to feel as though he/she is very important and special. Do not use professional jargon that the client may not understand.

19. I prefer to call people clients rather than patients. 'Patients' conjures up pictures of illness, hospitals and doctors.

20. Always have a good knowledge of other relative therapies; otherwise you will not necessarily recognise when another therapy may be more beneficial to the client. Never contact a doctor or another therapist without client's written consent.

21. Never treat beyond your skills. Never make false claims or promise cures. Be honest to yourself and others.

22. Whether working as a professional therapist or treating family do remember to record the oil used, the area treated, percentage of each oil used and the client's reactions.

23. All oil vapours are inhaled into the lungs no matter what the method of use.

24. The professional therapist will have learned through training the oils that should not be used in Aromatherapy and the various test methods used by the industry in an attempt to guarantee the quality of essential oils.

25. The professional therapist should have a double entry of all oils supplied to clients :
a. On the client record card
b. In a Sales Book kept specifically for this purpose.

26. Professional therapists must obtain client's written consent if it is his/her intention to contact the client's doctor.

27. HOMECARE oils should have recorded on the label: Purpose of oil, Safety instructions, Instructions for use, Date, Therapist's details, Telephone number, etc. (see page 73)

28. Therapist should be aware of what action to take in case of poisoning. (see page 52)

29. Therapist should be aware of how and when to do patch testing. (see page 52)

30. Therapist should be aware not to massage over areas of tumour or areas treated with radium treatment (the area should be kept dry).

31. Therapists should be aware that the reference "to avoid exposure to sun/sunbed after or prior to application of specific essential oils" infers that the area treated or to be treated should not be exposed and does not relate to those parts of the body not treated nor to be treated with essential oils.

32. Membership of lead organisations is the only way for the professional therapist to be sure of any changes or additions in the uses of essential oils brought about by research and discovery.

CONTRA INDICATIONS

DO NOT MASSAGE

1. Infected areas

2. When fever is present

3. When high temperature is present

4. For a couple of hours after a heavy meal (especially the tummy)

5   On an empty stomach (give a glass of fruit juice and a biscuit)

6. When the recipient is under the influence of either drugs or alcohol abuse

7   Undiagnosed pain (especially acute)

8   Unrecognised or undiagnosed skin conditions

9. Varicose veins (stroke only)

10. Area of swelling

11. Over areas of inflammation

12. Over a Fracture

13. Over a Bruise

14. Over a Hernia

15. Over Broken skin

16. Over Recent scar tissue

PRECAUTIONS

1. If in doubt always check with a Medical Practitioner

2. High humidity increases the permeability of the essential oil into the skin and therefore the client should be advised against having an Aromatherapy treatment prior to a further proposed treatment such as a turkish bath, sauna, steam bath or sunbed.

3. Make sure small children do not rub their eyes whilst having an Aromatherapy bath.

4. Do not use skin sensitising oils on clients with allergies, Asthma, Dermatitis, Eczema, Hayfever, Skin cancer or Melanomas.

5. Do not use citrus oils on skin cancer or melanoma patients.

6. Do not apply under the arms especially if any products other than washing soap is used.

7. Do not use perfumed products to cleanse skin prior to an Aromatherapy facial.

8. Do not use a strong mask on the face immediately prior to an Aromatherapy treatment.

Remember it is not within the skill of an Aromatherapist to make a medical diagnosis. That is the prerogative of the medically qualified or others recognised so to do.

BENEFITS OF MASSAGE

1. Human contact
2. Relaxes tight muscles
3. Improves vascular and lymph flow
4. Encourages the interchange of tissue fluid
5. Gives a general feeling of wellbeing
6. Total relaxation for mind and body

REASONS WHY YOUR CLIENT MIGHT NOT ENJOY THEIR MASSAGE

Bad breath
Offensive body odour
Tobacco or stale smell on body or clothing
Being unable to see therapist's face during the treatment (due to hair falling over face)
Breathing into the client's face
Client may not feel therapist has taken enough care with general hygiene
Nails too long and scratching client
Not allowing the client to relax (talking or playing loud music)
Getting facial cream or oil into client's eyes
Getting product on client's clothes
Getting product on client's hair unless that is the intention
Not helping client on to and off the couch
Not explaining treatment clearly, including the cost of the treatment
Not showing interest in the client's problem
Taking too long with treatment

ANALYSIS OF THE CLIENT'S FACE & BODY

SKIN

Check for :
Open pores, blackheads, whiteheads, oilyness, dryness, flakeness, rough texture, broken capillaries, eczema, psoriasis, athlete's foot, verrucas etc. bruising,blemishes, scars, pigmented areas,vitiligo, moles, muscle tone, hydration and dehydration.

On legs also check for:
Cellulite and varicose veins.

On arms also check for:
Cellulite.

Eyes:
Check if eyes are bright or lifeless and check if there are any dark circles.

Hair:
Check if the hair is dull and dry or bouncy and lustrous, is it fine or thick, is it sparse or plentyful, is it grey or is it well kept.

Posture:
Is it round and inward, is it upright and strong, is it slouched and relaxed or is it slouched and tense.

Check for:
Confidence/attitude
Full of confidence, confident (don't be fooled by the quiet client), shy, downtroden, aggressive, calm, relaxed or stressed.

SOME ASPECTS OF LIVING

The professional therapist can use this guide to expand his/her own inquisitive mind in order to give maximum benefit to the client in a practical and holistic way.

1. BREATHING

Problem - Why?
> Respiratory Illness
> Physical damage to the Respiratory System
> Common cold
> Asthma
> Heart condition

Look at the Cause
> Anxiety
> Emotional
> Stress
> Physical Conditions - Bad housing, Poor work environment,
> Self employed - Takes health risks, Heavy smoker

2. COMMUNICATIONS

Problem - Why?
> Physical disability
> Is he/she deaf
> Is he/she dumb
> Is it a difficulty to express feelings?

Look at the cause

> Hereditary
> Congenital
> Accident
> Illness e.g. malignant tumour
> Surgery
> Impaired mental development

Consider

> Can he/she use sign language or lip read?
> Can other family members use sign language or lip read?
> Is there frustration?

3. EATING AND DRINKING

Problem - Why?

> Mouth ulcers
> Recent digestive surgery
> Illness (Colitis, Crohn's disease, Ulcers, Anorexia)
> Compulsive eating disorders
> Alcoholic

Look at the cause

> Low income
> Poor housing - shared housing, effort to get to a cooker at
> meal times
> Disabled - cannot manage knobs and taps
> Not educated in nutritional values
> Low self esteem

Consider

> Other external or internal pressures

4. ELIMINATION

Problem - Why?
Digestive disease or illness?
Constipation or diarrhoea induced by anxiety or stress?
Urinary disease - cystitis, incontinence (double or single)?
Is it a bed wetting child?
Is the condition caused by external or internal factors?

5. CONTROLLING BODY TEMPERATURE

Problem - Why?
Elderly Person
Poor housing
Low income
Fear of spending money on fuel
Risk from hypothermia

Baby
External temperature too hot or too cold
Recognise the dangers - advise parents to
call doctor or ambulance if baby is showing signs for concern

Considerations
Is there a medical condition?
Should the sufferer see a doctor?

6. MOVEMENT

Problem - Why?
Temporary, due to joint sprain/strain or bone fracture
Is the condition psychosomatic?
Is it life threatening?
Is it degenerative?
Is it traumatic (car, bike accident) partially paralysed?

Considerations
Does he/she need referral to an Osteopath or Chiropractor?
Does he/she need hospitalisation, specialist services?

7. PERSONAL HYGIENE

Problem - Why?
Low income
Poor housing
Homeless
No bath
No hot water
Memory lapses
Mental impairment
Physical disability

8. SLEEPING

Problem -Why?
    Shift work
    Uncomfortable bed
    Noisy neighbours
    Physical pain
    Pressure of work
    Emotional problems

9. SEXUALITY

Problem - Why?
    Infertility
    Impotency
    Frigidity
    Illness/condition (Herpes, Thrush, AIDS)
    Emotional problems
    Physical problems

10. MAINTAINING A SAFE ENVIRONMENT

Problem - Why?

Low income	-	cannot replace damaged household equipment
Loss of smell	-	cannot detect smoke/fire
Physical disability	-	cannot mop up spillages
	-	unable to reach window catches, etc.

11. WORKING

Problem - Why?

    Mentally or physically unable to work
    High unemployment area
    Unemployment only temporary, due to accident
    Suffering with depression
    Housebound in wheelchair or has small children

12. DYING

Problem - Why?

    Grieving for lost partner
    Grieving for lost child
    Grieving for lost parent
    Terminally ill
    Nursing a terminally ill relative or friend

The therapist will explore the possibilities as to how he/she can help in these situations :

1. By referring the client to the appropriate professional person who can deal with a particular situation.

2. By making suggestions and offering information on societies and organisations which are able to help in certain situations, e.g. housing, grants, local authority counsellors or local organisations for the disabled.

3. The therapist should always have available an index box or book with the names and addresses of local complementary therapists and general professional organisations.

HINTS FOR RUNNING A SUCCESSFUL CLINIC

The therapist should have two index boxes on the desk.

Box one should contain - an outline of conditions, disorders, diseases, i.e. definition, usual symptoms, medical treatment. The back of the card should contain information such as a list of suitable oils and in red those oils that are contraindicated to that condition and the details of relevant precautions. This box could also contain details of societies and organisations not related to complementary therapy, e.g. Asthma Society, Epilepsy Society, etc. Two separate coloured cards could be used which make for ease of identification, i.e. white for disorders/diseases and blue for societies.

Box two should contain Names, Addresses and Telephone numbers of local complementary therapists from all fields and the back of each card should contain details of the relevant organisation. If recommending a therapist make sure you have visited that person to introduce yourself and feel happy with the response you received, (naturally you will leave your business cards/leaflets).

I have a third box on my desk, a small one containing information that will enable me to deal with almost any eventuality that might arise for myself or my client. In this box I have details of all local trades people, a mechanic, a locksmith, a baker and I also include the names of those that will do home visits. The AA and the RAC numbers have been useful to have on hand in the past as have the animal rescue organisations, when my clients have been ready to replace a departed pet. Sadly I also feel the need to keep details of the NSPCC.

Do not expect clients to remember details as they may be distressed by the time they require information from your little box. Therefore details should be written for them, preferably on the back of one of your own business cards.

I suggest you start your boxes when you start your business. Box one will act as a support and confirmation index especially in the early days of treating. Box two and three will be a source of referral which will save time when a client is present and will make you seem efficient and professional. It will also act as a means of advertising through the other local professionals and businesses on which you keep information .

SENCE OF SMELL
(What is the Human Olfactroy System?)

The scientific name for our sense of smell is Olfaction. Smell has in the past often been considered to be the least important of the senses yet it is probably one of the oldest and may well act more directly on our subconscious than any other.

Most of the nose is concerned with processing air flow on its way to the lungs. Only a very small part of the nose and nasal cavity is taken up by the organs of smell.

The organ of smell is a little yellow patch of olfactory epithelium (skin cells) located in the superior aspect of each nasal cavity. Each olfactory epithelium contains about five million olfactory receptor cells surrounded by support cells. The olfactory receptor cells are bipolar neurons, each with a thin dendrite that terminates in a knob from which several cilia (hair like structures) radiate.

According to the most common hypothesis, the olfactory receptor sites providing the interaction of odorants with olfactory receptors, are regions of the olfactory cilia outer cell membrane formed by glycoproteins. The cilia are covered by a coat of thin mucus produced by the olfactory gland (Bowman's Gland). These secretions keep the olfactory membranes moist and serve as a solvent for the odour molecules. The mucus contains odorant binding proteins which deliver odorants to the surface of cilia membranes where they bind with olfactory receptors, thus causing stimulation of olfactory neurons.

A few interesting facts about the olfactory system:

1. In order for a substance to be smelled it must be volatile.
   In other words it must be capable of entering into a gaseous state. It is these gaseous particles that enter the nostrils.

2. The unmyelinated axons of the olfactory receptor cells constitute the fibres of the 1st Cranial Nerve (Olfactory nerve).

3. Our sense of smell can distinguish thousands of chemicals, however research suggests that we have only between 15 and 30 kinds of receptors. These are stimulated in different combinations.

4. Pathway of Olfaction
    a. Fibres of the olfactory nerves synapse with mitral cells within the olfactory bulb.
    b. When mitral cells are activated impulses flow from the olfactory tract to the olfactory cortex where smell interpretation occurs.
    c. Olfactory tract fibres also project to the limbic area of the brain where emotional aspects of the smell are analysed. This area is closely related to the hypothalamus and is also the seat of learning, memory and emotion.

5. Breaths come in pairs, with the exception of twice in a lifetime. At birth we inhale for the first time. At death we exhale for the last time.

6. We breathe about 23,000 times a day. It takes approximately 2 seconds to inhale and 3 seconds to exhale.

7. Neurons in the nose are different to all others in the body in that they are replaced every few months. If neurons to the brain are damaged then the damage is permanant.

ANOSMIA

Those without sight are labelled blind, without hearing deaf. The loss of the sense of smell is known simply as anosmia. The complications and distress of such a condition are far reaching.

The loss of smell is usually the result of one or more of a number of factors. For example : Nasal cavity inflammation (caused by smoking, cold, flu), head injury, physical obstruction of the nasal cavity and olfactory mucus (e.g. polyp, genetic causes). Some brain disorders can have an effect on the sense of smell (e.g. epileptics sometimes find their sense of smell distorted).

The victim of anosmia loses not only the joy of being able to relive happy memories when receiving a luxurious rose oil massage but the smells of danger are no longer detectable (for example the smoke filled room). The treasures and pleasures of life so many of us take for granted are denied to this almost neglected group.

OLFACTORY FATIGUE

This is in a way a form of temporary anosmia. It mostly occurs when we smell the same odour continuously over a period of time. The nose is still able to detect other odours. Sensitivity to the original smell will return if the source of the smell is removed for a little while and then returned.

THE OLFACTORY SYSTEM

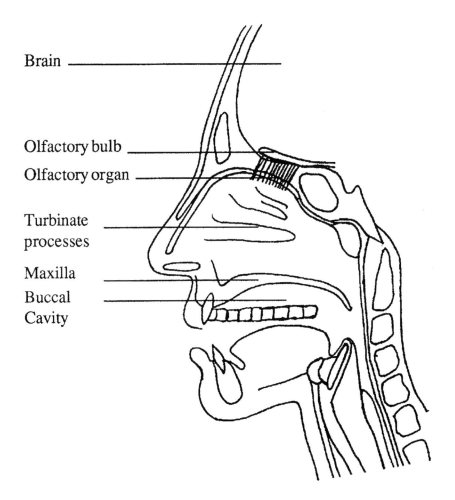

Brain

Olfactory bulb

Olfactory organ

Turbinate
processes

Maxilla

Buccal
Cavity

PREGNANCY

Essential Oils in PREGNANCY

It is worth commencing this section with the knowledge that no oils have been passed as safe to use in pregnancy. The normal term of pregnancy is nine months and is usually divided into three periods of three months each referred to as first, second and third trimester.

Pregnancy is a vulnerable time for mother and baby and the likelihood of a reaction to essential oils or for that matter to any drug therapy is enhanced, especially in those individuals who are less well nourished, are drug or alcohol addicts, smokers or suffer from chronic conditions such as diabetes.

It is well documented that certain drugs can cross over the placenta from mother to baby and I have no reason to believe anything different about essential oils. Small molecules pass into fetal circulation via the placenta and it is generally accepted that a substance with a molecular weight of 1000 can cross the placenta. Bearing in mind that essential oil constituents have weights below 500, it is most likely that they are capable of crossing the placenta. The blood brain barrier is not yet fully developed increasing the possibility that any components crossing the placenta will reach the fetal central nervous system. Because the system is still relatively underdeveloped it is more susceptible to damage by chemicals than the adult system.

The first trimester is the most critical period for the baby and in my opinion during this period it is best to avoid essential oils in massage other than commonly used citrus oils which are generally accepted in practise as being safe.

I tend to use only Mandarin and Tangerine during the first trimester. It is important to observe phytotoxicity guidance (keep out of the sun and off sunbeds before and after use for twelve hours) and also remember that the oils should be used only in low dilutions. I do not recommend the oils be used internally or via the vagina or rectum.

Other essential oils most commonly used in the massage practice for the

pregnant client are the gentle florals such as Chamomile, Geranium, Rose, Sandalwood and Lavender. Once again I would advise only very low dilutions (if at all) of between 0.5% and 1% maximum. Although these oils are used in practice many therapists will not use them in the first trimester.
Oils used for inhalation include Spearmint, Cajeput and Eucalyptus.

There are the obvious hazards in trying to study the effects of drugs, (or essential oils) in pregnancy. It is very difficult to predict which drugs may cause damage to the unborn child.

The observations of the damaging effects of drugs on pregnant animals does not always suggest similar effects on pregnant women.

LABOUR

Oils considered most suitable for using during labour are Clary Sage, Jasmine, Rose, Chamomile and Lavender. If considering using essential oils during labour do not bring a burner into the hospital as most delivery wards have oxygen cylinders on hand and the risk of accident is far too great.

A partner can massage back and lower abdomen with a pre-blended oil (best contained in a plastic bottle).

Some drops of oil could be inhaled from a tissue or dropped onto clothing. If the birth is at home the room could be sprayed with a pleasing scent.

AFTER DELIVERY

The following blends may be pre blended either by the therapist, or by the client at home

What you will need:

10ml	Evening Primrose Oil
10ml	Almond Oil
5ml	Vitamin E Oil (or two capsules)
6 drops	Lavender
4 Drops	Chamomile
2 Drops	Tea-Tree

Blend together and massage the perineum two or three times daily.

For Bath Soak

30ml	Almond Oil
6 drops	Lavender
6 drops	German Chamomile
3 drops	Tea-Tree

Blend together and add two teaspoons to the bath and have a ten minute soak. Take care not to slip when getting into or out of the oily bath.

If infection is present or after Episiotomy, change the recipe to the following:

6 drops	Lavender
6 drops	Tea-Tree
3 drops	German Chamomile

Blend together in 30ml Almond oil, add two teaspoons to the bath and have a ten minute soak. Take care not to slip when getting into or out of the oily bath.

SUMMARY OF THERAPEUTIC INDEX

Suitable oils and their method of use - Any one or maximum of three oils may be used in any one recipe for self help.
(See Blending Guide Page 66)

Abcesses
    Chamomile
    Eucalyptus
    Lavender
    Lemon
    Sandalwood
    Tea-Tree

Bath, Compress, Alcohol spirit

Abdominal Aches/Pains
    Chamomile
    Fennel - (Flatulence)
    Frankincense
    Marjoram
    Neroli
    Peppermint

Bath, Compress, Massage

Abrasions
    Frankincense
    Lavender
    Neroli
    Tea-Tree

Bath, Compress, Alcohol Spirit

Acne

Bergamot
Chamomile
Geranium
Juniper
Lavender
Melissa
Niaouli
Sandalwood
Tea-Tree
Thyme

Compress, Facial Steamer, Mask, Face lotion/cream

Addiction

Chamomile
Clary Sage
Jasmine
Neroli
Rose
Violet

Bath, Massage, Compress, Vapouriser

AIDS

Bergamot
Chamonile
Clary Sage
Jasmine
Lavender
Neroli
Niaouli
Rose
Tea-Tree

Bath, Massage, Compress, Vaporiser

Anaemia
>Chamomile
>Fennel
>Lavender
>Lemon
>Petitgrain
>Rosemary

Bath, Massage, Vaporiser

Anorexia
>Bergamot
>Chamomile
>Clary Sage
>Fennel
>Ginger
>Jasmine
>Lavender
>Neroli
>Rose
>Ylang-Ylang

Bath, Massage, Vaporiser

Anxiety
>Chamomile
>Clary Sage
>Frankincense
>Geranium
>Lavender
>Neroli
>Rose
>Sandalwood
>Violet

Bath, Massage, Vaporiser

Arthritis

Chamomile
Geranium
Ginger
Juniper - if swelling is present
Lavender - If condition is very painful
Marjoram

Bath, Massage, Compress, Vaporiser

Asthma

Bergamot	Immediately prior to or directly after
Chamomile	an attack try one of the following:
Clary Sage	
Cypress	Stay in moist area i.e. bathroom or
Eucalyptus	kitchen and add oil to water. Put the
Frankincense	drops of oil on hankie and inhale. I do
Lavender	not believe asthmatics should use
Marjoram	facial steamers at crucial times
Neroli	
Rose	

Bath, Compress, Vaporiser, Massage

Athlete's Foot

Lavender
Lemon
Niaouli
Tea-Tree

Bath, Compress, Cream, Spray

Backache
   Bergamot
   Chamomile
   Juniper
   Lavender
   Mandarin - mix with any of the above
   Myrrh
   Rosemary

   Bath, Massage, Compress

Bed Sores   (Pressure sores)
   Bergamot
   Chamomile
   Cypress
   Geranium
   Lavender
   Lemon
   Tea-Tree

   Compress, Cream, Spray

Bed Wetting
   Chamomile
   Lavender
   Mandarin

   Bath, Massage tummy and lower back, Vaporiser

Bilious Attack
   Chamomile
   Fennel
   Ginger
   Peppermint
   Rose

   Bath, Massage, Inhalation

Bites

> Chamomile
> Geranium
> Lavender
> Niaouli - Neat (one drop only)
> Tea-Tree

> Bath, Compress, Spray, Direct application

Bleeding

> Chamomile
> Cypress
> Geranium
> Lavender
> Lemon

> Compress

Blisters

> Chamomile
> Lavender
> Lemon
> Tea-Tree

> Spray direct, Cream direct, Ice cubes (wrapped in cloth)

Blood Pressure - High (Hypertension)

> Bergamot
> Chamomile
> Lavender
> Neroli
> Marjoram
> Rose
> Ylang-Ylang

> Bath, Massage, Compress, Vaporiser

Blood Pressure - Low (Hypotension)
    Bergamot
    Black Pepper 1%
    Jasmine
    Lavender
    Neroli
    Peppermint 1%
    Rose
    Rosemary

    Bath, Massage, Compress, Inhalation, Vaporiser

Boils
    Chamomile
    Lavender
    Niaouli
    Tea-Tree

    Bath, Hot compress

Bronchitis
    Cedarwood
    Cypress
    Eucalyptus
    Pine
    Tea-Tree

    Bath, Massage (chest and back), Vaporiser, Inhalation

Bruises
    Chamomile
    Fennel
    Geranium
    Lavender

    Ice Compress (ice wrapped in cloth)

Burns
>Lavender

>Cold water then neat application. Cold compress - apply oil regularly

Bursitis
>Chamomile
>Geranium
>Juniper
>Rosemary

>Bath, Compress, Massage (rest the affected area)

Candida Albicans (Thrush)
>Bergamot
>Lavender
>Lemongrass
>Myrrh
>Niaouli
>Tea-Tree

>Bath, Massage

Capillaries (broken)
>Calendula
>Carrot - blended
>Chamomile
>Cypress
>Rose

>Compress, Massage (gentle), Vaporiser

Catarrh
>Cedarwood
>Eucalyptus
>Lavender
>Lemon
>Tea-Tree

>Bath, Inhalation, Massage (throat, chest), Vaporiser

Coldsore - Herpes Simplex

Bergamot
Lavender
Tea-Tree

Neat - use damp cotton wool bud to apply

Colic

Chamomile
Fennel
Lavender

Bath, Abdominal massage

Colitis

Chamomile
Cypress
Geranium
Lavender
Neroli
Tea-Tree

Compress, Bath, Massage (gentle abdominal massage)

Constipation

Black Pepper
Fennel (sweet)
Juniper Berry
Peppermint
Rosemary

Bath, Abdominal massage (clockwise direction)

Corns
> Lavender
> Lemon

Local application, cover with a plaster during the day

Coughing
> Chamomile
> Cypress
> Eucalyptus
> Geranium
> Palmarosa
> Rose
> Tea-Tree

Bath, Inhalation, Massage (chest, throat, back), Vaporiser

Cramp - Leg
> Chamomile
> Cypress
> Geranium
> Rosemary

Bath, Massage, Foot bath (brisk rub)

Cramp - Abdomen
> Bergamot
> Chamomile
> Geranium
> Neroli
> Peppermint
> Rose

Bath, Massage, Compress

Cystitis
Bergamot
Chamomile
Eucalyptus
Juniper
Lavender
Sandalwood
Tea-Tree

Bath, Bidet, Compress, Massage (abdomen and lower back)

Dandruff
Chamomile
Cedarwood
Clary-Sage
Lavender
Patchouli
Rosemary
Tea-Tree

Lotion, Massage, Shampoo

Dental Abscess
Chamomile
Lemongrass
Myrrh
Niaouli
Tea-Tree

Massage cheek, Mouthwash with alcohol base.
Rub a piece of fresh Garlic onto the gum

Depression
Bergamot
Chamomile
Clary Sage
Jasmine
Neroli
Palmarosa
Violet

Depression (continued)
    Rose
    Sandalwood
    Ylang-Ylang

    Bath, Massage, Vaporiser

Dermatitis (patch test skin first before use)
    Bergamot
    Cedarwood
    Chamomile
    Geranium
    Juniper Berry
    Lavender
    Myrrh
    Neroli
    Rose
    Rosemary
    Sandlewood

    Bath, Massage, Compress

Diarrhoea
    Chamomile
    Cypress
    Ginger
    Lavender
    Neroli
    Peppermint
    Sandalwood
    Tea-Tree

    Compress, Gentle Massage (abdomen) - (reduce food intake)

Diabetes

Bergamot
Black Pepper
Eucalyptus
Geranium
Juniper
Lemon
Neroli
Rose

Bath, Massage, Vaporiser

Digestive Problems

Chamomile
Fennel (sweet)
Ginger
Lemongrass

Bath, Massage, Compress, Vaporiser

Diverticulitis

Bergamot
Chamomile
Eucalyptus
Marjoram
Peppermint
Tea-Tree

Bath, Massage, Compress

Energy Depletion

Bergamot
Geranium
Pine
Rose
Rosemary

Bath, Massage, Vaporiser

Fever
> Chamomile
> Lavender
> Peppermint

> Bath, Compress, Inhalation

Fibrositis
> Chamomile
> Cypress
> Juniper
> Lavender
> Rosemary

> Bath, Compress (alternate hot/cold), Massage, Vaporiser

Flatulence
> Fennel
> Ginger
> Mandarin
> Petitgrain

> Bath, Compress, Massage

Fleas
> Cajuput
> Eucalyptus
> Geranium
> Lavender
> Niaouli
> Patchouli
> Tea-Tree

> Bath, Local direct application

Frigidity
  Clary Sage
  Jasmine
  Rose
  Sandalwood
  Ylang-Ylang

  Bath, Massage, Vaporiser

Gallbladder - Stimulant
  Chamomile
  Lavender
  Lemon
  Peppermint
  Rosemary

  Bath, Compress, Massage, Vaporiser

Gout
  Chamomile
  Cypress
  Ginger
  Juniper
  Lavender

  Foot bath, Compress

Hangover
  Juniper
  Lavender
  Rose
  Rosemary
  Violet

  Bath, Head and abdominal massage, Vaporiser, Inhalation
  from tissue/hankie

Hayfever
  Juniper

  Vaporiser, Inhalation from tissue/hankie

Headaches
  Chamomile
  Juniper - Allergy
  Lavender - tension
  Peppermint
  Rose - Allergy
  Rosewood

  Bath, Compress, Vaporiser, Massage

Herpes Zoster
  Chamomile
  Eucalyptus
  Geranium
  Lavender
  Tea-Tree

  Bath, Compress, Vaporiser

Hoarseness
  Cedarwood
  Eucalyptus
  Lavender
  Sandalwood

  Massage, Vaporiser, Inhalation from tissue/hankie

Hot Flushes
Rose
Chamomile
Geranium
Clary Sage

Bath, Massage, Vaporiser, Inhalation from tissue/hankie

Hypertension   See page 292 (High) Blood Pressure

Hypotension   See page 293 (Low) Blood Pressure

Indigestion
Chamomile
Peppermint

Bath, Compress, Inhalation from tissue/hankie, Abdominal
massage (clockwise)

Impotence
Clary Sage
Jasmine
Peppermint
Rose
Sandalwood
Violet
Ylang-Ylang

Bath, Massage, Vaporiser

Insomnia
Chamomile
Lavender
Mandarin
Marjoram
Ylang-Ylang

Bath, Massage, Vapouriser

Kidney Problems
Bergamot
Cedarwood
Fennel
Frankincense
Geranium
Juniper
Sandalwood

Bath, Compress, Massage

Lice
Eucalyptus
Geranium
Lavender
Tea-Tree

Head massage/shampoo, Hair spray

Ligaments - Painful
Lavender
Lemongrass
Rosemary

Bath, Local massage, Compress

Liver
Chamomile
Juniper
Lemon
Peppermint
Rosemary

Bath, Hot/Cold compress

Lymphatic System
Fennel
Geranium
Grapefruit
Juniper
Rosemary

Bath, Massage. **DO NOT** give lymphatic drainage massage to patients suffering with Cancer or Aids or any serious condition of the autoimmune system.

Menopause
Bergamot
Chamomile
Geranium
Jasmine
Lavender
Neroli
Palmarosa
Rose
Sandlewood
Violet
Ylang-Ylang

Bath, Massage, Compress, Vaporiser

Memory
Basil
Lavender
Lemon
Peppermint
Rosemary

Bath, Massage, Inhalation

Metabolism - Sluggish
Juniper
Lavender
Lemon
Peppermint
Pine
Rosemary

Bath, Massage, Vaporiser

Migraine
Chamomile
Cypress
Fennel
Lavender   (Most analgesic oils will help)
Lemon   **NOTE!** - Smells might exacerbate
Marjoram   an attack.
Peppermint

Bath, Compress, Self massage around temples (very light)

Mosquitoes
Eucalyptus
Geranium
Lavender
Lemongrass
Niaouli
Patchouli

Bath, Spray body (in alcohol or lotion base)

306

Multiple Sclerosis (M.S.)

Bergamot
Chamomile
Geranium
Jasmine
Juniper
Lavender
Neroli
Peppermint
Rose
Rosemary

Bath, Massage, Compress, Vaporiser

Muscle Aches

Black Pepper
Chamomile
Juniper
Lavender
Marjoram
Rosemary

Bath, Massage, Compress

Myalgic-Encephalomyelitis (M.E.)

Chamomile
Geranium
Grapefruit
Lavender
Neroli
Niaouli
Palmarosa
Rose
Sandalwood
Tea-Tree

Bath, Compress, Inhalation, Vaporiser

Nappy Rash
> Chamomile
> Lavender
> Vitamin E oil
> Wheatgerm

Bath, Cream (see "Recipe" section page 332)

Nausea
> Chamomile
> Ginger
> Lavender   - With migraine
> Neroli
> Peppermint   - Travel sickness

Bath, Abdominal massage, Inhalation, Vaporiser

Neuralgia
> Cajuput
> Chamomile
> Lavender
> Peppermint

Compress, Gentle massage, Vaporiser

Nettle Rash
> Chamomile
> Lavender

Cold compress, Cool bath

Obesity

    Bergamot
    Fennel
    Geranium
    Grapefruit
    Jasmine
    Orange
    Rose
    Sandlewood

    Bath, Massage, Diffuser, Inhalation from tissue/hankie

Palpitations

    Chamomile
    Clary Sage
    Lavender
    Neroli
    Rose
    Ylang-Ylang

    Bath, Massage, Vaporiser

Periods - Heavy

    Cypress
    Geranium
    Rose

Periods - Painful

    Chamomile   **CHECK** with your GP and
    Lavender   then with a professional
    Marjoram   therapist
    Violet

Periods - Scanty, Late

Clary Sage
Fennel
Juniper
Rose (regulator)
Rosemary

DO NOT use essential oils
if there is a chance you
might be pregnant. See your GP

Baths, Compress, Massage abdomen and lower back

Perspiration

Cypress
Geranium
Lavender
Rose

Bath, Foot bath, Massage, Alcohol-based spray

Premenstrual Syndrome

Bergamot
Chamomile
Clary Sage
Fennel
Geranium
Lavender
Marjoram
Neroli
Rose
Ylang-Ylang

Bath, Massage, Compress, Vaporiser, Inhalation

Psoriasis
Bergamot
Chamomile
Eucalyptus
Frankincense
Juniper
Lavender
Rose
Sandalwood

Bath, Local Compress, Vaporiser

Respiratory Weakness
Cypress
Eucalyptus
Lavender
Peppermint
Rosemary
Tea-Tree

Bath, Massage, Compress, Inhalation, Vaporiser

Rheumatism
Bergamot
Chamomile
Juniper
Lavender
Marjoram
Neroli
Niaouli
Pine
Rosemary

Bath, Compress, Massage

Rubella
> Bergamot
> Chamomile
> Cypress
> Eucalyptus
> Lavender
> Sandalwood
> Tea-Tree

> Bath, Compress, Vaporiser

Sinusitus
> Cypress
> Eucalyptus
> Lavender
> Tea-Tree

> Inhalation, Vaporiser, Facial Massage

Sprain (joint)
> Black Pepper
> Chamomile
> Eucalyptus
> Ginger
> Lavnder
> Rosemary

> Compress

Strain (muscle)
> Bergamot
> Chamomile
> Clary Sage
> Geranium
> Neroli
> Rose
> Sandalwood

> Bath, Massage, Vaporiser, Inhalation

Tension

Bergamot
Chamomile
Clary Sage
Jasmine
Lavender
Marjoram
Neroli
Rose
Violet

Bath, Massage, Vaporiser, Inhalation

Tonsilitis

Chamomile
Geranium
Lavender
Palmarosa
Tea-Tree

Bath, Vaporiser, Inhalation

Toothache

Chamomile
Lavender
Niaouli
Tea-Tree

Massage cheek, Mouthwash solution in alcohol base.
Rub a clove of Garlic on gum.

Urinary Infections
Bergamot
Cedarwood
Eucalyptus
Tea-Tree
Sandalwood

Bath, Bidet, Compress, Massage, Vaporiser

Varicose Veins - Legs
Cypress
Geranium
Lemon

Bath, Massage (very gentle stroking towards heart)

Varicose Veins - Haemorrhoids
Chamomile
Cypress
Lemon

Bath, Bidet, Lotion/Cream

Viral Conditions
Eucalyptus
Lemon
Melissa
Tes-Tree

Vaporiser, Local application, Inhalation

Water Retention

Cypress

Fennel

Geranium

Grapefruit

Juniper

Bath, Massage, Compress

Wounds (Infected)

Chamomile (German)

Frankincense

Lavender

Myrrh

Niaouli

Palmarosa

Tea-Tree

Compress - wash/soak, Direct application - spray

POTENIALLY HAZARDOUS ESSENTIAL OILS
NOT TO BE USED IN AROMATHERAPY

Almond Bitter
Armoise
Artemisia
Arborescens
Basil
Birch
Boldo
Buchu
Cade
Calamus
Camphor (brown)
Camphor (yellow)
Cassia
Cinnamon bark
Costus
Elecampane

Fig leaf
Horseradish
Lanyana
Mustard
Penny Royal
Sage (dalmation)
Sassafras
Snake root
Tansy
Tarragon
Tea
Thuja
Verbena
Wintergerm
Wormseed
Wormwood

MASSAGE OIL RECIPES

MASSAGE OILS RECIPES FOR SPECIFIC CONDITIONS
BLENDED IN 25 ml CARRIER

Anxiety/Depression
4 drops Clary Sage
2 drops Patchouli
4 drops Ylang-Ylang

Apathy/Anxiety
4 drops Grapefruit
4 drops Lavender
4 drops Rosemary
or
4 drops Neroli
4 drops Lavender
2 drops Lemon

Extreme Nervousness
3 drops Clary Sage
3 drops Jasmine
4 drops Bergamot

Irritability
2 drops Petitgrain
4 drops Sandalwood
4 drops Chamomile

Relaxing Oils
4 drops Rose
2 drops Tangerine
or
8 drops Lavender
4 drops Chamomile
or
8 drops Marjoram
4 drops Chamomile

Spasticity
Local Massage of area
6 drops Ginger
6 drops Lavender
or
6 drops Cypress
6 drops Chamomile
or
6 drops Rosemary
4 drops Sandalwood
2 drops Chamomile

Stimulating Oils
8 drops Rosemary
4 drops Bergamot
or
8 drops Rosemary
4 drops Grapefruit

BATH OIL RECIPES

Blend bath oils prior to putting into bath. Use either carrier oil, alcohol, non oily bath emulsion or a non perfumed foam bath. I blend 3 drops of essential oil to every 5ml (approximately one teaspoon) of carrier. The first time of using the oil put 5ml into the bath and if you are happy with the outcome you could use 10ml (6 drops) of oil thereafter.

Aphrodisiac Bath
2 drops Sandalwood
1 drop Ylang-Ylang
or
1 drop Sandalwood
1 drop Neroli

Wake-Me-Up Bath
am or pm
2 drops Rosemary
1 drop Geranium
or
1 drop Peppermint
1 drop Rosemary
1 drop Geranium

Fluid Retention/Cellulite
1 drop Geranium
1 drop Juniper
1 drop Sweet Fennel
or
1 drop Juniper
1 drop Sweet Fennel
1 drop Cypress

Insomniac Bath
1 drop Clary Sage
2 drops Chamomile

Total Indulgence Bath
1 drop Rose
1 drop Mandarin
or
1 drop Jasmine
1 drop Mandarin
or
1 drop Neroli
1 drop Geranium

TIPS FOR AN AROMATIC BATH and SHOWER

BATH

Prepare your bath in the normal way and when half full add the prepared oil mixture and swish it around with your hand, (remember to keep the doors and windows shut so as not to lose any of the vapour). Do not have the water too hot as it is bad for your skin and don't have it too full that you can't add more hot water as the bath cools.

A fifteen minute soak would be sheer luxury (bring a good book) but even a ten minute soak will make a real difference.

SHOWER

Prior to getting into the shower prepare the mix as for the bath but instead of bath oil use a non perfumed shower gel.

Add 10ml (2 teaspoons) of the prepared mix to a large sponge and place this onto the shower floor. Begin to shower as normal. When your body is really wet rub the sponge all over your body but taking care to avoid your eyes, then shower again. An alternative way to use the mix would be to shower or bath as normal and then use the mix as a body lotion. However only two drops should be used to each 10ml of non-perfumed lotion for this purpose, especially if for use more than twice a week.

NOTE !

Use a maximum of 6 drops of essential oil to any bath or shower, irrespective of the amount of base or carrier used.

Remember to try 1 teaspoon of the mix first time. If there are no adverse effects to the oil then add 2 teaspoons in the next bath or shower (2 teaspoons refers to prepared blended mix and does not mean pure essential oil). Essential oil may be added to a non perfumed shower product in much the same way as for bath use.

GENERAL PRODUCT RECIPES

GENERAL BASE CREAM/OINTMENT

What you will need:

105ml	Grapeseed
50ml	Wheatgerm or suitable alternative oil
20 grams	Beeswax
175 drops	Essential oil

A large saucepan
A tall pyrex or metal jug
A spatula or long handled spoon
Some small pots / jars

If you would like a softer cream make the following blend:

70ml	Grapeseed
55ml	Wheatgerm or suitable alternative oil
25 grams	Beeswax
25 grams	Vaseline - or instead of Vaseline use 10ml Rose Water and 15ml Glycerine
175ml	Add to this mixture 175 drops of oil

NOTE ! Vaseline offers a protective external film.

How to prepare your mix :

Prepare a large saucepan of water and place on a heating element of a stove. Into this stand a tall jug-type pyrex or stainless steel container.

1. Add the wax to the jug

2. When wax has melted reduce the heat under the saucepan

3. Add all other ingredients, apart from the essential oil

4. Leave saucepan on the stove and stir the mix together. Do not allow the mix to boil

5. Turn off the stove and carefully remove the jug from the water

6. Wait for the mix to begin to cool and set

7. The setting/cooling shows around the edge of the jug first

NOTE ! If wax is grated it will melt faster.

Pour the contents of the jug into individual pots and stand these pots in a tray of cold water so they are submerged to between one third and half their height. Alternatively surround the pots with ice. This action speeds up the cooling process.

As the mix cools the essential oil should be added. Different essential oils could be blended for each pot but remember to mix acurate and even amounts. Seal the pots wipe dry and label.

This cream should last for about a year, especially if a clean cotton wool bud is used each time some of it is removed.

NOTE!
Use for localised conditions only, eg. sprains/strains, athlete's foot, boils, frozen shoulder, acne spots on the back, etc.

SKIN CARE GUIDE

Suitable Oils for Home Preparation

Dry Skin

Rose
Chamomile
Sandalwood
Neroli
Frankincense

Oily Skin

Rose
Rosemary
Lavender
Grapefruit
Geranium

Mature Skin

Rose
Neroli
Frankincense
Sandalwood
Ylang-Ylang

Acne

Rosemary
Juniper
Lavender
Tea-Tree
Geranium
Violet

Sensitive Skins

Rose
Chamomile
Lavender

Very Sensitive Skins

Use no more than
1 drop to 10ml
Carry out patch test if worried

For specific conditions see pages 287 to 315 or read the appropriate oil profile.

NOTE !
I do not reccomend Juniper or Rosemary oils to be used on the face.

CLEANSING CREAM

What you will need:
    60ml Almond oil
    60ml Rosewater
    15 grams Beeswax
    10 drops essential oil
- large saucepan
- tall pyrex or metal jug
- spatula or long handled spoon
- rotary whisk or fork
- some small pots/jars

Method of preparation:

Put a large saucepan half full of water onto the heating element of a stove, into this stand a tall pyrex or stainles steel jug.

Place the wax and Almond oil into the jug and wait for the wax to melt (grated wax will melt quicker). Turn off the source of heat. Remove the jug carefully from the saucepan.

Slowly add the Rosewater while using a rotary whisk or a fork. Continue to add slowly and whisk until all the water has been absorbed (do not overbeat). When it is cool add the essential oil to the mix, then stir all the ingredients together; the handle of a long spoon can be used if a clinic spatula is not available.

Empty the mix into small individual pots and stand them on a tray, surround each pot by ice. If no ice is available then put cold water in the standing dish/tray, When cool, seal, wipe dry and label clearly. Now place the pots in a cold place; they should keep for about six months to one year if kept very cool and not contaminated with fingers or a dirty spatula.

SKIN TONIC

What you will need:
200ml	Bottle
80ml	Orange flower water or Rosewater
80ml	Filtered tap water or distilled water
10ml	Alcohol (Vodka)
16 Drops	Essential oil

For a very oily skin use 20ml vodka / 70ml water.

Method of Preparation:
Blend oil into vodka
Pour into 200ml bottle
Add floral water
Add pure water
Label bottle
Turn bottle up and down about 10 times. Shake gently each time before use.

AFTERSHAVE

What you will need:
200ml	Bottle
150ml	Orange flower water
15ml	Vodka/Alcohol
10 drops of	Essential oil

Most suitable oils are Sandalwood, Bergamot, Cypress and Frankincense.

Method of preparation is as for Skin Tonic

SKIN MOISTURISER / CREAM RECIPE

What you will need :

60ml	Almond oil
7 grams	Beeswax
15ml	Distilled water
2ml	Vitamin E oil
8 Drops	Essential oil

A large saucepan
A tall pyrex or metal jug
A spatula or long handled spoon
A rotary whisk or fork
Some small pots / jars

Method of preparation is exactly the same as for the Cleansing Cream. Page 323

NOTE !

If skin is very dry or mature the moisturiser can be altered in one of two ways:

1. Instead of 60ml Almond oil use 30ml of Almond oil and 30ml of Avocado oil plus 1ml of Evening Primrose oil.

or

2. Use 60ml of Jojoba oil instead of Almond or Avocado plus 1ml of Evening Primrose oil.

Mixture 1 or 2 would be suitable to use as a night cream or neck cream.
Should keep for about one year if kept in cool conditions and not contaminated by fingers or dirty spatula.

SHAMPOO RECIPE

Purchase a natural shampoo such as Chamomile. To each 100ml add a maximum of 10 drops of essential oil. Use the shampoo in the normal way. A total of two oils are recommended with the maximum being three oils.

Hair care index guide:

Dry Hair	Oily Hair	Dandruff
Sandalwood	Rosemary	Rosemary
Geranium	Juniper	Tea-Tree
Rose	Bergamot	Eucalyptus
Ylang-Ylang	Clary Sage	Lavender
	Lemon (if blonde)	

HEAD LICE SHAMPOO RECIPE

Purchase a natural shampoo such as Chamomile. To each 100ml add 50 drops of essential oil. Use the shampoo in the normal way. A total of two oils is recommended with the maximum being three

The oils to use

Eucalyptus
Geranium
Lavender
Patchouli
Tea-Tree

Wash alternate days for one week and then twice per week for two weeks. Use a special fine-tooth comb after washing (available from chemists)

AN ALTERNATIVE REMEDY

Mix any two of the above oils into one tablespoon of carrier oil. Massage into the hair and leave for half an hour. Then wash and fine-comb hair. Repeat the following day and again one week later.

NOTE !
Be careful to keep this mix away from the eyes.

To remove oil apply a mild shampoo and massage in before applying water.

MOUTHWASH RECIPE

What you will need:
>250ml Bottle (plastic for the bathroom)
>250ml Vodka/Alcohol
>20 Drops of Thyme
>10 Drops of Tea-Tree
>10 Drops of Fennel
>10 Drops of Peppermint

How to prepare your mix:
>Add Vodka/Alcohol to the empty bottle
>Add essential oil

How to apply:
>Add 15ml (approx. 3 teaspoons) of your mixture to half a tumbler of water
>Use as normal mouthwash

NOTE !

Do Not swallow the mixture and remember to shake bottle before each use

HAND AND NAIL CARE RECIPE

What you will need for basic preparation:

50ml	Bottle
25ml	Avocado oil
25ml	Grapeseed oil
	Essential oil
	Cotton wool buds

(1)) Cracked Brittle Nails	**(2) Bitten Nails and Skin**
add	add
20 drops Lemon oil	10 drops Lavender oil
	5 drops Lemon oil
	5 drops Chamomile oil

Add the avocado, grapeseed and essential oil to the bottle and shake the bottle to mix ingredients. Apply all over the nail twice daily using a cotton wool bud.

Dry Hands

Use basic preparation as for Nails but use the following essential oils. This preparation would be massaged into the hand (no cotton wool bud required).

5 drops	Geranium
5 drops	Chamomile
2 drops	Rose
or instead of Rose use	
5 drops	Frankincense

Nail Fungus

20ml	Vodka
12 drops	Tea-Tree
2 drops	Lavender

Apply three times each day using a cotton bud or wear protective gloves avoiding direct contact with the affected nail.

ATHLETE'S FOOT RECIPE

What you will need:

Recipe one (a cream)
50ml pot of bland cream
1 vitamin E capsule
20 drops Tea-Tree
(alternatively 10 drops Tea-Tree and 10 drops Myrrh)
20 drops Lemon or Lavender (especially if skin is broken)

Recipe two (a spray)
100ml of Vodka in a plastic bottle with spray attachment
20 drops Tea-Tree oil
20 drops Myrrh
10 drops Lavender

Mix all the ingredients together.
Massage into feet twice a day wearing disposable gloves for this routine to avoid spreading infection.
Spraying recipe is a more hygienic method of application and can reduce the risk of spreading the infection.

NOTE !
The essential oil mix should not be kept in a plastic bottle for longer than four weeks due to the risk of possible chemical interaction.

VERRUCA

What you will need :
    20ml bottle with either Vodka or Jojoba oil
    1 Vitamin E capsule
    6 drops Lemon
    6 drops Tea-Tree
    2 drops Lavender

Mix the ingredients together.
Apply directly to the area twice daily using a cotton wool bud or wear a pair of disposable gloves. Cover with a plaster during the day but remove the plaster at night and do not replace the plaster after the evening treatment.

Do persevere - this preparation may take a little longer to do its job than some 'over the counter' chemicals.

NOTE !
The essential oil mix should not be kept in a plastic bottle for longer than four weeks due to the risk of possible chemical interaction.

SWEATY FEET RECIPE

What you will need :
    100ml bottle with either Vodka or Jojoba oil
    20 drops Lemongrass
    20 drops Cypress
    10 drops Tea-Tree

Mix the ingredients together and massage feet daily.

NOTE !
The essential oil mix should not be kept in a plastic bottle for longer than four weeks due to the risk of possible chemical interaction.

NAPPY RASH RECIPE

FIRST AID

Prepare a general base cream/ointment. (see recipe on page 320)

To 175ml of the base cream/ointment add

> 5ml of either Jojoba, Avacado or Calendula
> 30 drops of essential oil = 18 of Lavender, 12 of Chamomile

If you do not have the facilities to follow the recipe on page 320 purchase a bland cream from the chemist and to each 175 ml of cream add the 30 drops of essential oil as above.

REGULAR - NAPPY CHANGE PREPARATION

As for 'Nappy Rash' but increase the quantity of base/carrier to 250ml and keep essential oil at 30 drops maximum.

If using washable nappies add 2 drops of Lavender to a bucket of rinse water or 4 drops to the fabric softener in your washing machine.

NOTE !
Essential oil might colour/stain plastic.

ROOM SPRAY / AIR FRESHENER / INSECT REPELLANT

What you will need:

100ml	Plastic bottle with spray top
20ml	Vodka
80ml	Water
20 drops	Essential oil

How to prepare your mix:

Add Vodka to the empty bottle
Add 20 drops essential oil
Add the water
Put the cap onto the bottle and shake vigorously

Air Freshner

To create a clean, fresh smell use Lemon or Cypress.
For floral smells use Ylang-Ylang, Sandalwood or Geranium.
For flu/cold use Eucalyptus, Tea-Tree, Lavender, Cypress

Insect repellant

Ants, Fleas, Flies, Moths, Mosquitoes, Ticks and general insects.
Cajuput, Cedarwood, Geranium, Lavender, Lemongrass, Niaouli,
Patchouli, Peppermint, Tea-Tree, Thyme.

Method of use:

Spray area of habitat.
Hang some ribbons soaked in essential oil from the curtain rail.
Put cotton wool pads soaked with essential oil in the area of problem.

BE AWARE GUIDE

Undiluted Oils
Generally speaking undiluted oils are not used in massage, neither are they used on diseased or broken skin, eyes, cuts, wounds or mucous membrane. The main reason for this is to avoid inflammation.

There may however be times or situations when it might be considered by some that the benefits of such action may outweigh the risk, such as bites, burns, herpes simplex (cold sore), herpes zoster (shingles), malignant ulceration, leg ulcers, verrucas or warts. In the more serious conditions medical supervision would be strongly advised.

Alcoholics
I do not advise oral consumption of essential oils by anyone and it is especially important that this rule is observed by alcoholics.

Allergies
Those prone to allergies related to fragrances may well be allergic to essential oil. Men are 2½ times more sensitive to irritation than women and Orientals tend to be more sensitive to skin reactions than Europeans.Changes of season - October and March may trigger sensitivities in those prone to allergies and sensitivities.

Baths
Modern baths may be stained by essential oils.

Breast feeding
Avoid the following oils : Lemongrass, Fennel, Melissa and Geranium. Use oils in low dilutions and ensure no oil is on the nipple. If oils used in a mixture to help cracked nipples remove traces of oil by using a carrier oil followed by lots of warm water before putting the baby onto the breast. Babies are attracted to their mothers smell and this could be affected by the use of essential oils.

Cancer or skin exposed to radiation
Do not massage directly over the area of tumour or site of treatment.

Children
Under one year old do not use essential oils in a bath or massage and thereafter use in very low dilution 0.05% to a maximum of 1%.
Children and babies are very sensitive and may well react. Keep away from eyes and never give children essential oils orally.
Add Chamomile tea bags to a bath (take care that they are not sucked by the child) or add waters of Rose or Orange flower.

Compress
Mix essential oil in carrier to avoid any possible skin irritation.

Douching
Mucous membranes are very sensitive to essential oils and irritation is likely unless the oil is preblended. Essential oils are difficult to disperse in water.

Driving
Clients may become very relaxed during an Aromatherapy treatment or after a long soak in the bath which could lead to disorientation. Ensure the client is wide awake before they attempt to drive or operate machinery.

Eyes
Essential oils should not be used on or near the eye.

Migraine
Use essential oil with great caution during an attack as strong odours may exacerbate an attack.

Patch Test
Patch test all new oils especially if skin sensitive or prone to allergies of any kind.

Peppermint
Do not use in the bath, may cause skin reactions.

USEFUL TERMS EXPLAINED

1. **Acute**
    Short and severe, not long drawn out or ongoing.

2. **Carcinogenic**
    An agent capable of inducing cancer.

3. **Chemotype**
    The same plant grown in different regions and under different conditions can produce essential oil of diverse characteristics.
    For example : The chemical composition of Rosemary (Rosmarinus Officinalis) can vary according to whether grown at the coast or inland. Spanish Rosemary containing a high amount of Borneol is call Chemotype Borneol. African Rosemary is called Chemotype Cineole due to its relatively high Cineole content.

4. **Chronic**
    Lasting, ongoing.

5. **Decoction**
    A herbal preparation made by boiling the plant material for 10-20 minutes, starting with cold water.

6. **Essence**
    A substance which naturally occurs within a plant.

7. **Herbal Oil**
    An oil prepared by steeping the plant material in a bland oil.

8. **Idiosyncratic Sensitisation**
   An abnormal reaction to a normally harmless substance. In other words it is an individual reaction rather than perhaps one of the more common reactions such as allergy to metal.

9. **Infusion**
   A herbal preparation made by pouring boiling water on the fresh or dried herb (as for teas).

10. **Irritation**
    Dermal/Cutaneous irritation refers to the effect on the skin indicating that the chemical has been absorbed and the cells are reacting against it, resulting in reddening and swelling.

11. **LD50 (Lethal Dose)**
    The lethal dose which kills 50% of the animals tested is the number of grams which is related to the body weight of the animal. Relative to man 10g/kg is equivalent to 700g per 70kg. Long term effects can manifest themselves 1-30 years after a person has been subjected to small doses of chemicals.

12. **Maceration**
    A herbal preparation made by steeping the plant material at room temperature for hours or days. The liquid may be water, alcohol, wine or oil.

13. **Mutagenesis**
    A substance or agent that can produce genetic mutation.

14. **Organic Chemicals**
    Organic is accepted in general meaning as a substance
    that is natural and untampered with. In chemistry the
    word organic means "containing the element Carbon".
    All essential oils and vegetable oils are mixtures of
    chemically organic molecules.

15. **Phototoxicity**
    Refers to reactions of skin that is exposed to ultra violet
    light after the application of essential oil or chemicals.

16. **Photoallergenic**
    Is the response of an organism to a substance causing
    allergic sensitivity to light. Some oils possess phototoxic
    properties but generally tend not to be photoallergenic.

17. **Sensitisation**
    Simply means allergic reaction. An intense form of
    irritation involving the immune system. Even small
    amounts of the offending agent can cause severe
    reactions. Manifestations of reactions are usually
    dermatitis or local swelling. A severe reaction can be
    anaphylactic shock which causes general collapse,
    affecting breathing and blood pressure and can be fatal.
    Caution ! Once sensitized to a chemical, even a related
    chemical can cause similar reactions. This is an important
    factor in Aromatherapy.

18. **Teratogenic**
    Effects are seen only in next generation. Parents
    having had no toxic symptoms after exposure to
    chemicals.

19. **Tincture**
A clear liquid prepared by macerating the plant material in alcohol, pressing and finally filtering.

20. **Toxicology**
The study of poisoning - In relation to essential oil this could be taken to mean allergic, cancer, phototoxicity, pregnancy and skin irritation, etc. Factors taken into account are age, state of health, blood pressure, organ function/disfunction, especially the liver and kidney.

21. **Trace Elements / Constituents**
The proportions of certain trace elements are so minute that they have to be expressed as so many parts per million or even trillion. Yet these infinitesimal amounts can sometimes be detected by the human nose and in some cases they can completely characterise the odour of the essential oil.

Quality Control of Essential Oils

1. **Gas Liquid Chromatography (GLC) Analysis**
    A piece of equipment used in the laboratory to
    separate the vapour of a volatile mixture into its
    individual components. The results of the GLC are
    printed out by an instrument onto a sheet of paper as a
    series of peaks with each peak corresponding to one of
    the constituents of the product being analysed. For
    accuracy the results of the GLC analysis must be
    interpreted by an expert in the field.

2. **Mass Spectrometer**
    An instrument coupled to the GLC, which breaks up
    into fragments the molecules of the individual
    constituents of the products from which the analyst can
    identify a constituent.

3. **I.R. Spectrophotometer**
    An infra red instrument which gives a graph
    reflection of the composition of the material being
    tested. Each essential oil has its own characteristic
    print. Like human fingerprints each essential oil
    print is individual, being different from those of
    any other essential oil.

NOTE !
Only very specialised techniques using cyclodextrins can show
adulteration with synthetics. Such adulteration may well go
undetected due to time and expense.

USEFUL ADDRESSES

Aromatherapy Organisations Council (A.O.C)
P.O Box 19834
London
SE25 6WF
England
Tel / Fax: 020 8251 7912

Associationof Aromatherapists of South Africa
PO Box 23924
Claremont
Cape Town. 7735
South Africa

The Atlantic Institute of Aromatherapy
16018 Saddlestring Drive
Tampa
FLORIDA 33618
USA

Federation of Holistic Therapists
3rd Floor, Eastleigh House
Upper Market Street
Eastleigh
S050 9FD
Tel: 023 8048 8900

International Examination Board (I.E.B.)
1 Northumberland Avenue
Trafalgar Square
London. WC2N 5BW
England
Tel : 020 7872 5456

International Federation of Aromatherapists (I.F.A)
182 Chiswick High Road
London. W4 1PP
Tel: 020 8742 2605

USEFUL ADDRESSES

International Society of Professional Aromatherapists (I.S.P.A)
ISPA House
82 Ashby Road
Hinckley
Leicestershire. LE10 1SN
Tel: 01455 637987

Irish & International Aromatherapy Association
Roscore
Blueball
Tullamore
C0. Offaly
Eire

ITEC Professionals
10/11 Heathfield Terrace
Chiswick
London. W4 4JE
Tel: 020 8994 7854

Register of Qualified Aromatherapists (RQA)
PO Box 3431 Danbury
Chelmsford
Essex. CM3 4UA
Tel: 01245 227957

Renée Tanner Lecturing
Acorn House
Cherry Orchard Road
Croydon
Surrey. CR0 6BA
England
Tel: 020 8686 4781

Index

C

D

E

F

G

H

I

347